VIBRANT HEALTH
The Ultimate Weight, Heart, And Health Program

by
Dr. Clifford T. Stewart, Ph.D.
and
Dr. Lawrence A. Fehr, Ph.D.

TOP OF THE MOUNTAIN PUBLISHING
Largo, Florida 34643-5117 U.S.A.

Top Of The Mountain Publishing
11701 South Belcher Road, Suite 123
Largo, Florida 34643-5117 U.S.A.
SAN 287-590X
FAX (813) 536-3681
PHONE (813) 530-0110

Copyright 1993 by Dr. Clifford T. Stewart /
Dr. Lawrence A. Fehr

Library of Congress Cataloging in Publication Data
Stewart, Clifford T.
Vibrant Health: The ultimate weight, heart, and health program/by Clifford T. Stewart and Lawrence A. Fehr.
p.cm.
Includes bibliographical references, glossary, and index.
ISBN 1-56087-015-X (trade pbk.): $12.95
ISBN 1-56087-071-0 (hard back): $22.95
1. Reducing. 2. Nutrition. 3. Health. I. Fehr, Lawrence A. II. Title.
RM222.2.S82 1993 613.2'5—dc20   91-28265CIP

Manufactured in the United States

DEDICATION

To Goldie, Diane, David, and Linda Stewart.

To Kathy, Jason, and Ryan Fehr.

ACKNOWLEDGMENTS

We wish to extend to our wives, Goldie Stewart and Kathleen Fehr, our gratitude for their help, understanding, and forbearance as we gave our time and energy to this book.

To Sue Murray, whose consistent good humor sustained her and astounded us as she typed countless versions of each chapter, we offer our enduring thanks.

We wish also to thank our editors, Yvonne "There's a more recent study" Fawcett, who made sure that we considered the latest research before we wrote any conclusion, and Joe "Scissorshands" Straub who truncated and translated our abundant, abstruse, and arcane professional jargon into a concise book that can be read in something less than a lifetime.

FOREWORD

The optimal physical and mental health of its people should be society's highest priority. However, this can only come about when a country's citizenry demands it. We believe that this decade offers promise in this area the likes of which have never before been witnessed in recorded history.

This belief is based on four important points. First, research conducted by physicians, psychologists, dietitians, physical therapists, and other health professionals has conclusively proven that lifestyle factors have a major impact on physical and mental health. This has helped people realize that they do have some power over their current and future state of mind and body. Second, an increasing number of people in the Western world have taken this power and become active participants in their own wellness. Third, the media have become more interested in health issues — which has led to a more knowledgeable populace who demand action from government and industry. Fourth, the corporate world has begun to realize that money can be saved through wellness programs. All of these facts have made us truly enthusiastic about the future of individuals and their goal of achieving "Vibrant Health!"

One negative side to this current interest is that many of the diet and other wellness programs put on the market in recent years are based on gimmicks and fads rather than on the ever-increasing body of scientific knowledge. Too many books and tapes tell people what they want to hear rather than what they should know. It is our position that wellness involves disciplined and ongoing efforts in nutrition, exercise, and stress reduction — that wellness cannot rely on short-term solutions or miracles.

We are encouraged by the recent ground breaking efforts of Dr. Dean Ornish, assistant clinical professor of medicine and an attending physician at the School of Medicine, University of California, San Francisco. His research has shown that a very strict program of nutrition, exercise, and stress reduction can actually *reverse* arterial blockage caused by cardiovascular disease. Our program, not as strict as that of Dr. Ornish, is designed to help those millions of people who are not already battling with an advanced disease; those who wish to avoid ever entering that battlefield.

We call our program VIBRANT HEALTH because it is designed to take our readers beyond what they have experienced or perhaps even imagined, to the utmost they can achieve for their bodies and minds. By following the scientifically-based principles in this book, you will improve your chances of living a longer, richer, much happier life. Here's to you and your VIBRANT HEALTH!

Clifford T. Stewart, Ph. D.
Lawrence A. Fehr, Ph. D.

DISCLAIMER

The information in this book reflects current thinking and practices at the time of writing. Because of ongoing research, practices and recommendations may change.

This book is intended as a reference volume only, not as a medical manual or a guide to self-treatment. If you suspect that you have a medical problem, we urge you to seek competent medical help. Keep in mind that needs (nutritional, exercise, etc.) vary from person to person, depending on age, sex, and health status. Information here is intended to help you make knowledgeable decisions about your life, not to be substituted for any treatment that may have been prescribed by your doctor.

TABLE OF CONTENTS

Table of Contents

CHAPTER 1

EATING YOUR WAY TO HEALTH

"CODE BLUE !!!!! — Room 402"
Ten minutes later . . . .
"WE'VE LOST HIM!"

Those are words which we hope never to hear. They pertain to our fictitious (but in many ways typical) patient, Jack Robertson, who has just suffered his second heart attack. Unfortunately, this one was fatal. Could it have been avoided?

Obviously, there are no guarantees in life. You may be physically fit and still be struck by lightning tomorrow, but why make life's gamble greater than it already is? Was it anything Jack Robertson did that made his gamble greater than it had to be?

Jack did not live a terribly unusual life. As a boy, he was successful academically, but disliked sports and other physical activity. He spent most afternoons and evenings reading or watching television, accompanied by his two constant companions — potato chips and chocolate chip cookies. When he was in high school, his father died of a heart attack at age 45. This upset Jack tremendously, and his response was to ease his sorrows through increased food intake. About this time, Jack also began to smoke.

In college, Jack was an honor student, and after graduation, he was hired by a major accounting firm. His pre-employment physical showed that his blood pressure was 150/94. His physician recommended that he decrease his salt intake, quit his three-pack-a-day smoking habit, and try to shed 100 of the 286 pounds he carried around on his 5'10" frame. Jack assured his doctor that he would try.

As an accountant, Jack was extremely success-ful. He passed his C.P.A. exam at age 25, and by the time he was 32, his 18-hour work days landed him a controller position in a large firm. A workaholic, Jack had little time for other pursuits. He married his college sweetheart and fathered three children in rapid succession but spent little time with them. Vacations were nonexistent and he was rarely home for dinner. At 40, Jack's insurance physical uncovered a blood pressure of 162/105, a cholesterol level of 341, and a weight of 301 pounds. The physician made numerous recommendations, and placed Jack on hypertension medication which he took sporadically — whenever he happened to think of it.

Jack suffered his first heart attack at the age of 44. It was discovered that he had several blocked arteries necessitating a quadruple heart bypass. Unfortunately, Jack thought of the surgery as a cure for his condition, so he failed to change his lifestyle in any significant way. He suffered his fatal heart attack four years later at the age of 48.

At this point, you may feel relieved that your situation is not as desperate as Jack's. But his lifestyle can be broken down into many component parts, which many of us share — each of which was hazardous to good health.

EATING YOUR WAY TO WELLNESS

It was clear from Jack Robertson's profile that his health and dietary habits were less than ideal. In order to help you avoid Jack's fate, we will focus on a nutritional strategy you can adopt to prevent obesity, hypertension, and high cholesterol — and even to help you limit your risk of heart disease, stroke, and cancer. This sounds like high hopes and a big order — but you'll find that the same basic eating strategy will help with *all* of these health problems.

DON'T DIET

That's right. You should never "go on a diet." The problem with a diet is that most people think of it as something you "go on" with the ultimate goal of eventually "going off." A genuinely helpful "diet" is never a short-term attempt — it is an *eating plan for the rest of your life*. Obviously, people who are at immediate health risk may need to adopt drastic dietary restrictions for fast results, but that represents a very small part of the population.

For the rest of us, our goals should be to understand what is in the foods we eat and what they can do for us, and to gradually modify our eating habits. *Gradual* change is important, if you are to make the kinds of changes that you will be willing to follow for the rest of your life. Deprivation and starvation are simply not beneficial or realistic. You will not be willing or able to "deprive" yourself for the rest of your life. If you feel deprived, you will be miserable. Being miserable can make you ill. Being miserable can make you crave fats and sweets.

You want to combine physical health with emotional health — and the best way to do that is not deprivation but KNOWLEDGE. If you learn more about the foods you eat — their ingredients and their effects upon you — then your dietary improvement is just around the corner.

IS IT REALLY A "WEIGHT" PROBLEM?

Many people, particularly young females, repeatedly go on needlessly strict diets. The first question you should ask yourself is, "Do I really have a weight problem?" What is the ideal weight for you? The correct answer is that there is no "ideal weight." You should take your ideal weight charts and trash them. They support the mistaken notion that the quality of your physical condition depends on your weight — and that your goal should therefore be to eat less so that you will weigh less. This is wrong.

Even though most people lose weight when they improve their dietary habits, you should not think of your condition only in terms of pounds or kilograms. For example, Hershel Walker, who gained fame as a member of the Minnesota Vikings football team, has been tested and found to be "ideal" in terms of conditioning, nutrition, and health. Mr. Walker weighs approximately 230 pounds — and would be labeled overweight by almost any weight-height chart. So scrap the charts, and concentrate on health.

The problem with focusing upon pounds gained and lost is that we don't know what has been gained or lost. For example, I weigh more after drinking several pints of water, but that has nothing to do with my physical condition.

FAT IS THE ANSWER

If weight is not the best index of physical condition, then what is? The answer is FAT. The most important goal for most people who believe they have a weight problem should be to *reduce their body fat*. How can you determine your percentage of body fat? How will you know if a "diet" has resulted in a decrease or an increase in your percentage of body fat?

To consider the second question first, you can easily determine whether you are gaining or losing fat by the old-fashioned method of watching how your clothes fit. But the wrong kind of diet can actually cause you to gain fat and lose muscle, even while you are losing weight.

Take, for example, Jim Davis (not his real name). During a three-month recuperation for a broken leg and several other injuries from a car wreck, Jim ate a great deal of the wrong (high fat) foods and engaged in no physical activity. He was pleasantly surprised that he didn't gain any weight, until he discovered that his waist had increased two inches.

He had lost muscle from inactivity, but his unhealthy eating habits had increased his body fat. Since *fat weighs less than muscle*, he gained no net weight, but his physical condition and health clearly deteriorated. The extra two inches around his waist were not water or muscle, but fat.

Jim should be particularly concerned because recent research has shown that *all fat is not equally damaging*. It is *upper body* fat around the waist that *increases risk of heart disease* and other problems. This is a greater contributor to heart disease in men than in women, since men are more likely to store fat in the abdominal region. Women tend to accumulate fat more easily on the hips and thighs. The common terms for these body shapes are "apple shape" and "pear shape," respectively.

How can you determine your percentage of body fat and evaluate whether or not it is excessive? The most sophisticated method, performed at some hospitals, can give an exact measure of body fat by placing you in a tank of water and measuring the amount of water displacement. If two people weigh the same, the one with more fat will displace more water, since fat and muscle displace water differently.

A second and less sophisticated method involves the use of skin calipers, to measure the amount of fat that can be "pinched" at particular points on the body. This estimate can be done at many health spas, sports rehabilitation facilities, and hospitals.

If you do not have access to either of these two techniques, you can make use of Tables 1-A and 1-B to approximate your percentage of body fat. The tables are accurate enough to establish a base-line of your current physical condition, which you can use to chart your progress on your road to WELLNESS.

Sample Body Fat Percentages for MALES

Weight	Waist Measurement	Percent Body Fat
160	34	20
	36	24
	38	28
	40	34
180	34	17
	36	21
	38	26
	40	30
200	36	18
	38	22
	40	26
	42	30
220	36	16
	38	20
	40	24
	42	28
240	38	18
	40	22
	42	26
	44	30

Table 1-A

Sample Body Fat Percentages for FEMALES

Height (inches)	Hip Measurement (inches)	Percent Body Fat
60	34	22
	36	26
	38	30
	40	34
62	34	21
	36	25
	38	29
	40	33
64	36	24
	38	28
	40	32
	42	36
66	36	22
	38	26
	40	30
	42	34
68	36	21
	38	25
	40	29
	42	33

Table 1-B

Notice that for men, it's weight versus waist measurement; for women it's height versus hip measurement. *For men, a reasonable goal is 15-19% body fat; for women, 21-25% is fine.*

Keep the following points in mind:

✳DO focus on body fat.

✳DO attend to the way your clothes fit.

✳DON'T focus on weight charts.

✳DON'T use pounds lost as the sole means of monitoring your physical condition.

✳DON'T weigh yourself daily. It will give you a false sense of failure or success. Once a week is enough.

PATHWAYS TO SELF-IMPROVEMENT

Book stores carry countless "Diet Books" which suggest everything from high protein diets to no-carbohydrates diets to single-food diets to eliminating-certain-basic-food-groups-for-a-large-part-of-the-day diets. And someone is bound to think of a limiting-fluid-intake-on-alternate-Thursdays diet! These "fad" diets are the bad news about health and nutrition today. The often-contradictory information presented in them has led to mass confusion. Worse, they lead many of you to view yourselves as failures because you have followed one or more of these diets and still don't look like an aerobic instructor.

But the good news is that in the last several years significant strides have been made in the science of nutrition, based on studies around the world that have produced consistent scientific evidence. It is the significance of this evidence which has led to the suggestions made in this book.

Since we now know what works, why don't most people follow these guidelines and why aren't all diet books written with these guidelines in mind? Perhaps the most honest answer lies within the character of our population. We are an impatient society of doers who want results NOW.

Legitimate experts will not promise to let you take off 50 pounds in six weeks. In fact, a rapid weight loss of this magnitude would have long-term negative consequences for most of you.

The term "weight loss" has become part of our culture. But realize that when you say, "I lost a pound today," you unconsciously want to find that little pound tomorrow. So, remember that real weight loss means weight that you take off and LEAVE off — a *permanent* weight reduction.

Our strategy focuses on *losing fat and maintaining muscle*. And it opposes any program which severely restricts the number of calories you eat daily (except in extreme cases as directed by your physician). Our strategy emphasizes a modest weight loss of 1-2 pounds per week — by building habits that you will want to maintain for the rest of your life. Unfortunately, saying that you will never be able to return to your old eating habits is about as popular as a politician promising to raise your taxes. But the best news is that if you CHOOSE good-tasting, nutritious food, you won't WANT to return to your old ways.

Let's assume you are overweight, mildly hypertensive, and with an elevated but not disastrous cholesterol level. What should be your strategy? Basically, you should accept nutritional guidelines which will gradually improve your condition. Whether your concern is your waistline, your weight, your cholesterol level, or whatever, a series of easy short-term goals works best.

For example, if your waist is 45 inches, set a goal of reducing it to 43 inches. Once that is achieved, set a second goal of 41 inches, and so on. The advantage to this is clear. If you were to focus exclusively on your long-term goal of 34 inches, the task would be overwhelming, and you would be more likely to give up.

To attain each of your short-term goals, you will simply cut down your caloric intake. We are not proposing calorie counting. Never. But rather, we suggest adopting a basic sound nutritional strategy of eating meals with the proper balance of complex carbohydrates, protein, and a little fat. This strategy allows you to easily, painlessly adjust your eating habits in order to accelerate fat loss — even if you hit one of those famous "plateaus."

Of course, the true secret of success in your overall strategy must be to combine balanced nutrition with a consistent program of *aerobic exercise* — defined as any vigorous exercise that conditions the heart and lungs by increasing intake of oxygen to the body. This will help raise your metabolic rate even more — thus optimizing your body's ability to burn the calories that you take in during the day.

And, of course, you will need to improve your knowledge of the components in the food you eat.

For example, did you know that an average ounce of potato chips has 10-20 times the fat content of an ounce of pretzels? This is the kind of information which helps you make healthy changes with minimal sacrifice. Our goal is to show you how to decrease the percent of your body weight that is made up of fat, and increase the percent that is muscle.

CHAPTER 2

KNOW WHAT YOU ARE EATING

What should we eat and how much? The easiest way to remember this is to refer to the *Agriculture Department's pyramid* (Figure 2-1). After much controversy and many delays, the pyramid emerged as the victor over other visuals (including the pie, the wheel, the bowl, a shopping cart, food on a table) as the best way to portray the newly recommended diet.

What does it tell us? In brief, it says to eat more grains, fruits and vegetables, and eat less fat and

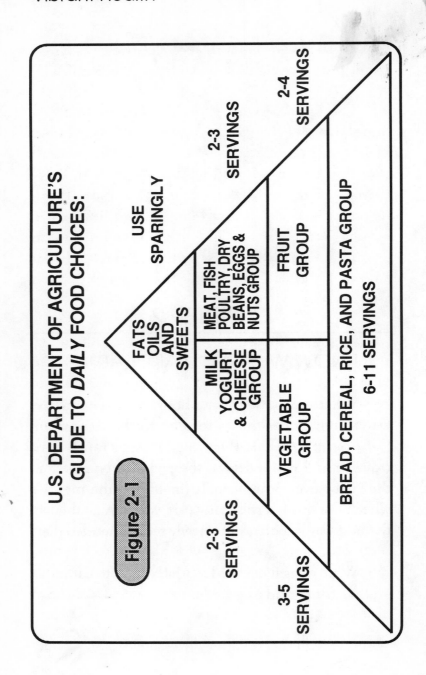

U.S. DEPARTMENT OF AGRICULTURE'S
GUIDE TO *DAILY* FOOD CHOICES:

Figure 2-1

USE SPARINGLY

FATS OILS AND SWEETS

2-3 SERVINGS

MILK YOGURT & CHEESE GROUP

MEAT, FISH POULTRY, DRY BEANS, EGGS & NUTS GROUP

2-3 SERVINGS

3-5 SERVINGS

VEGETABLE GROUP

FRUIT GROUP

2-4 SERVINGS

BREAD, CEREAL, RICE, AND PASTA GROUP

6-11 SERVINGS

sugar. You already knew that? Well, strange as it may seem, most people didn't. And they still don't.

The U.S. Department of Agriculture (USDA) hopes that will change, and so do we. This pyramid of the food groups will become the model for modern nutrition education. You will be seeing it in every newspaper and magazine article on nutrition. It will be on television. It is not only the latest, it will also be long-lasting. The USDA spent about a million dollars in deciding on this particular graphic (from among 400 tested), and that's not going to happen again very soon.

Now, after all the brain power, time, and money spent coming up with this pyramid (which was finally accepted in April, 1992) there is still controversy. Some of it comes from interest groups representing various foods on the pyramid chart, and some from those with no vested interests, but they have concern that this is not the best visual. So be it.

We also have one concern, which is that the top of the pyramid, unlike all the other sections, does not represent a food group. You don't go into a restaurant and order a bowl of fat, a serving of sugar, and a small glass of oil! These products are contained *in* the foods in the other five groups; fats and oils occurring more in the two food groups just below the top of the pyramid (milk, cheese, meat, poultry, eggs). Vegetables also contain oils — but with the exception of palm oil and coconut oil, which are highly saturated and not at all recommended — vegetable oils are necessary in a balanced diet. Sugars naturally present in raw fruits are no problem, but sugars added to processed fruits should be kept to a minimum.

Sugar substitutes are used by millions of people because they contain fewer calories than sugar. A packet of *Sweet'N Low*® (manufactured by Cumberland Packaging Corp.) contains four calories while sugar, to provide the same sweetness, would provide 30 calories. On the negative side, this product contains saccharin which has been found to cause cancer in laboratory animals. Its possible effects on humans are not fully known. The second popular artificial sweetener, *Nutrasweet*®, and *Equal*® (both manufactured by NutraSweet Co.) is actually *aspartame*, which has been reported to cause headaches, blindness and other symptoms, in some users. This is probably caused by a limited ability in these individuals to metabolize *phenylalanine* which forms the basis for this sweetener. If you have any such symptoms, stop using the artificial sweeteners for two weeks and see if the symptoms disappear.

In place of food or drink that use sugar substitutes, we recommend items sweetened naturally with fruits and fruit juices. These cookies, muffins, etc. produced by several companies, including *Health Valley*, can be purchased in health food stores. However, even if you shop in health food stores, it is still important to read labels because the nutritional properties of foods sold in these stores do vary.

Don't think that you are eating a healthy diet just because you don't choose anything from the top of the pyramid. Understand that this portrayal is to emphasize that fats, oils, and sugars should be kept to a minimum. And you do that by keeping to a minimum your food choices from the next level down (such as milk, cheese, meat, poultry, and eggs; and from any foods with sugar added). *In general, graze freely in the bottom of the pyramid and the next level up, but don't stretch for the third level too frequently.*

How do we go about applying these nutrition principles to our daily lives? Most packaged foods sold in stores list the ingredients, the number of calories per serving, plus the number of grams of fat, protein, and carbohydrates. Read those labels. To maximize your ability to burn the calories you eat, we suggest the following ratio:

60-65% of your calories from COMPLEX CARBOHYDRATES — fruits, vegetables, whole grain breads and cereals, nuts and seeds, beans and pasta. Avoid simple sugars — ice cream, candy, cake; and avoid all white bread products. (Remember that story about the lab rat that died after a diet of white bread? And that old solution to your ant problem — feed 'em white sugar?)

15-20% of calories from PROTEIN — yes, a big reduction. It's part of the International Revolution at the Food Front — instead of a *meat* being the main course, it's now only a *side dish*. The best sources are low-fat dairy products, fish, skinless white-meat poultry and lean meats. (Hot dogs and cold cuts are now on the most unwanted list!)

15-20% from FAT — mono-unsaturated olive oil, and polyunsaturated sunflower oil, safflower oil, corn oil, or canola oil. More about all these later. Remember that some fat is necessary for a healthy body, skin, hair, and nails — some, not much.

Follow these new percentages listed above. Other recommendations — 10% fat, for example, as proposed by Dean Ornish (in his book, *Dr. Dean Ornish's Program for Reversing Heart Disease*) — are unrealistic for happy lifestyle eaters.

This percentage breakdown is based on the fact that *all calories are not handled similarly by your body.* COMPLEX CARBOHYDRATES provide you with a source of *sustained energy* as well as *maximum calorie burn.* They are the fuel which ignites and speeds up your metabolic fire. PROTEIN is important to keep your body from using existing muscle as an energy source while you are burning carbohydrate calories. This decrease in muscle would in turn decrease your metabolic rate, and decrease the burning of your fat.

Average Westerners get about 40% of their calories (double the recommended amount) from fat. These fat calories hinder optimal calorie burn, and it is the excess fat calories that are most easily stored in your abdomen or hips. *The decrease in fat is the most needed change in your eating habits* — and also the most difficult to accomplish for many.

How do you know how many fat calories you ingest daily? You can calculate the amount from any packaged food that lists fat content. And several books list the fat content in a wide range of foods. Thus, you can calculate the percentage easily. *Each gram of fat contains 9 calories,* so if you are eating out and have a double cheeseburger, large order of fries, and vanilla milk shake, you have eaten 70 or more fat grams and are thus getting more than 60% of that meal's

Excellent Sources of Complex Carbohydrates, Protein, and Fat

COMPLEX CARBOHYDRATES Column A	PROTEIN Column B	FAT Column C
Fresh fruits (except avocados and coconut)	Chicken or Turkey (white meat, no skin)	Low fat cottage cheese
Fresh vegetables (green, yellow, red)	Beans (pinto, navy, lentils, garbanzo/chick peas, baked beans)	Skim or 1% milk No fat or low fat yogurt
Pasta	Egg whites (whole egg — no more than four a week)	"Lite" cream cheese
Semolina		
Whole grain breads pumpernickel bagels	Tuna (packed in water)	"Lite" mayonnaise (sparingly)
Potatoes with skins	Cheeses (low fat)	Mono-unsaturated oil
Cereals (high fiber only)	Lean red meat or pork (1-3 small servings per week)	Polyunsaturated oil
Popcorn (no oil)		
Pretzels (unsalted)	Fish (cod, flounder, haddock, halibut, mackerel, salmon)	Table 2-A
Brown or Wild rice		

calories from fat! This is far more fat than you should consume in an entire day.

In your new lifestyle, you will be eating fewer and fewer packaged goods, canned goods, frozen dinners — and more fresh fruits and vegetables.

> *Your nutritional goals should be to maximize your intake of complex carbohydrates, to minimize your intake of fat, to keep a moderate level of protein intake and generally, to limit the calories you consume. This overall strategy will help speed up your metabolic rate, decrease your percentage of body fat, control blood pressure and cholesterol, and protect your body against muscle loss. All of this will work best when diet is combined with aerobic exercise.*

On the next page are listed some commonly available high-quality sources of complex carbohydrates, protein, and fat. (Table 2-A)

Your discerning mind will notice much crossover in these foods — vegetables, rice, even fruits have protein (how else could vegetarians be so glowing with health?). Meats and dairy, of course, each have fat as well as protein. Nature is not an all-or-nothing designer.

WHAT YOU SHOULD BE EATING: DAILY ALTERNATIVES TO "HIGH-CAL"

Rather than give you specific menus, our approach is to give you alternatives — health-giving CHOICES — to beat back your desire for high fat and simple-sugar foods. This will give you a successful weight-reduction and fitness program. Obviously, if you want to lose weight you should also *be light-handed with your portions*. And learn to recognize your body telling you that you've had enough.

*DO avoid eating during the last three to four hours before bedtime. Your *metabolism is slow at night*, still slower while you're sleeping off that midnight snack.

*DO perform at least 20-30 minutes of aerobic exercise three or more times per week, as described in detail in Chapters 4 and 5.

Although we realize that most of our medicines come from plants, we don't regard food as medicine. In the Eastern part of the world (China, India, Japan), food has long been regarded as medicine. In parts of these countries, your treatment for illness might include specially selected foods, and perhaps herbs, roots, and leaves. As scientific medicine has

DAILY MEAL ALTERNATIVES
**You may substitute with similar items.
These are just examples.**

BREAKFAST
Choose One from Each Column

A (mostly carbohydrates)	B (carbohydrates)	C (protein and fat)
1 bare bagel with no-sugar jam (just as sweet)	1 banana	1 cup skim or 1% milk
1 cup hot cereal (high fiber)	1 orange	
1 cup cold cereal (high fiber)	1 peach	1/2 cup low fat cottage cheese
1 English muffin (whole wheat, pumpernickel)	1/2 grapefruit	
1 oat bran or whole wheat muffin	1/2 cup pineapple or berries	1/2 cup low fat yogurt
1-2 slices of bread (whole wheat, oat bran, alfalfa sprouts)	small glass of orange or grapefruit juice	
1 waffle (low-cal syrup)	small glass of cranberry juice	Table 2-B
1 buckwheat pancake (with fresh fruit, low-cal syrup)	small glass of tomato or V-8 juice	
	1/2 cantaloupe or 1/4 honeydew	

Vibrant Health

LUNCH

Choose One Each from Columns
A, B, and C; and Two from Column D

A
1-2 slices whole
wheat bread

1/2 cup brown rice

2 bread sticks

1/2 baked potato

1 bagel

B
**Choose from Column B
in Breakfast**

C
3 oz white meat
chicken or turkey

3 oz tuna fish
(water-packed)

1/2 cup low fat cottage
cheese

3 oz broiled, steamed
or baked flounder,
cod, haddock, salmon

D
(1/2 cup of 2 choices,
1/3 cup of 3 choices)

1 cup carrots

1 cup beans

1 cup cabbage
(green, red, Chinese)

1 cup broccoli,
brussel sprouts or
cauliflower

1 cup green leafy —
kale, spinach,
mustard greens

1 cup rutabaga or
yellow turnip

1 cup any kind of
squash

1 cup beets

Table 2-C

40

progressed in the Western world, we have forgotten the cures used even by our great-grandparents. *We are what we eat. What we eat becomes us.*

Let's discuss "high fiber" and "low fiber." The cereals screaming at you from the supermarket shelves and over the TV are not high fiber — they are *processed*, which by definition removes their fiber. Bran flakes are not whole grain, so *Total, Special K,* and other cereals are processed and punched up with added vitamins — but are *not* high fiber. HIGH FIBER means *unprocessed*, whole grain. Whole bran does have some fiber, but the *best* for you are the *rolled cereals — rolled oats, oatmeal, and especially, granola.*

Granola by any brand name is still rolled oats, and it is one of your body's best cholesterol-busters, as well as one of the primary high fiber foods. Try loading it with yogurt and fresh fruits (including berries) and milk. Now, *there's* a breakfast. The Swiss even have it for a light and very healthy evening meal.

```
┌─────────────────────────────────────┐
│                                      │
│              DINNER                  │
│                                      │
│   Same as lunch with the exception   │
│    that you may choose only one      │
│           from column D.             │
│                                      │
│          ( Table 2-D )               │
│                                      │
└─────────────────────────────────────┘
```

Do you love berries, melons, all kinds of fruit? That "choose one" (in the Breakfast Table 2-B) means *at least* one. It's even better to enjoy a medley — but, of course, cut your portions. The same is true for vegetables — the more kinds the merrier. Mix and match. Eat raw or cooked. And always try to have one yellow vegetable (which contains beta carotene) with the green.

Be sure you have salads — many salads of rich dark green lettuce or spinach, onions, parsley, celery, radishes, tomatoes. Or you may serve an antipasto tray of these. Don't forget the olives.

Also, and most important — the given portion of "one cup" of vegetables is *maximum*, unless you are large-boned and very active. For most of you (especially if you are small-boned with a small stomach) stay under one cup. Bon appetit!

Remember to snack on fruits, and even raw vegetables. They help keep you away from those high-calorie content foods.

One additional note about fruits and vegetables — some nutritionists tell us not to mix them (the fruits & vegetables) together. You may, therefore, wish to eat fruit 1/2 - 1 hour before your meals, or 3 - 4 hours after your meals. Veggies, of course, are eaten as part of your meal (or as a snack).

You don't want to give up butter? There is a compromise for those of you who feel you can't live without it. Follow the "recipe" of that famous nutritionist, Adelle Davis. In your blender, mix a half pound of butter (sweet, no salt) with a half cup of health-food-store blend oil (soy, safflower, sunflower, canola, walnut). This blend oil contains lecithin and Omega-3 — and like olive oil, actually helps to break down the cholesterol which would build up in your blood if you ate butter alone.

Vitamins are extremely important to your health. This isn't a vitamin book but a short course here might be helpful. More information on vitamins can be found in Chapters 10 and 11, where we talk about reducing your risk of heart disease and cancer. The first five vitamins in the alphabet constitute a very important group.

Vitamin A is necessary for healthy skin and bones (including teeth and gums), and for good vision. It helps us to resist infections, including colds, and strengthens our natural immunity.

Vitamin A can be found most abundantly in liver, followed by sweet potatoes, carrots, spinach, cantaloupe, broccoli, squash, apricots, and watermelon.

The B vitamins include B-1 (thiamine), B-2 (riboflavin), B-3 (niacin/niacinamide), B-6 (pyridoxine), and B-12.

This group of vitamins will give us energy, strengthen the nervous system, repair tissue, help form antibodies and red blood cells, and improve concentration and memory.

These vitamins are found in soy beans and wheat germ (B-1), kidneys and liver (B-2), beef liver and tuna (B-3), bananas and salmon (B-6), and beef liver (B-12). If you hate liver, get a good book on vitamins (see Bibliography), and discover the other foods that are rich sources of these and other vitamins.

Vitamin C helps us resist infection, speeds healing and detoxifies potentially harmful chemicals that our bodies produce and those chemicals that we eat. Oranges, grapefruit, papaya, brussel sprouts, and broccoli are the best sources.

Linus Pauling, the only person to win two unshared *Nobel Prizes*, has written for many years about the virtues of vitamin C, concentrating on its ability to stave off and to lessen the effects of the common cold, and, in fact to do the same for cancer. The U.S. recommended daily allowance (U.S. RDA) for vitamin C is 60 milligrams. Linus Pauling believes that this amount is enough to prevent scurvy, but is not enough to promote good health. He believes, after decades of research, that we would all benefit from taking from 6 to 18 grams or more each day (6,000 to 18,000 milligrams). He takes 18 grams daily.

In December, 1991, Pauling was diagnosed with prostate cancer and was asked whether he had changed his mind about the protective effects of vitamin C. He replied that the vitamin C might have put the cancer off by 10 years, and that practically all old men have some stage of prostate cancer sooner or later (Pauling turned 91 years old in 1992).

Also in 1992, a study at UCLA showed that 150mg daily of C extends life expectancy in men by two years, and 300mg increases it by six years. Pauling's 1986 book, *How to Live Longer and Feel Better*, may have a more accurate title than medical science has been prepared to admit.

Vitamin D is necessary for strong bones. It is found in fish liver oils and egg yolks. It is also produced when the sun hits our skin and converts a form of cholesterol into vitamin D.

Vitamin E protects us from heart disease. Increasing evidence points also to a role in enhancing the immune system and defending against infectious diseases. Wheat germ oil and sunflower oil and seeds supply vitamin E.

HYPERTENSION AND CHOLESTEROL REMINDERS

If you follow the suggestions in this and other chapters, you will begin to gain CONTROL of body fat, weight, cholesterol, and hypertension. (If you take hypertension medication, do not reduce it or stop taking it without consulting your physician.) To lessen your cholesterol levels, hypertension, even your risk of cancer — make the following DOs and DON'Ts part of your nutritional future — starting today:

✳DO eat three meals per day, at scheduled times; skipping meals just makes you hungrier; eat your larger meal at midday, not in the less-active evening.

✳DO use mono-unsaturated olive oil, or poly-unsaturated oils; limit saturated fats; and avoid palm and coconut oils.

✳DO cut mayonnaise by adding an equal amount of yogurt.

✳DO eat oat bran, wheat brans, and other high fiber foods; increase your intake of fruits and vegetables.

✳DO eat broiled, steamed, or baked fish.

✳DO use lean cuts of meat; limit your intake of red meat, and cut down your portions of all meats.

✳DO limit your intake of cheese — and then make it low fat, low sodium.

✳DO limit eggs to four or fewer per week.

✳DO read ingredient labels.

✳DO choose low fat snacks such as popcorn (air popped), and pretzels.

✳DO exercise regularly.

✳DO limit your consumption of alcohol, and switch from "hard" liquor to moderate amounts of red wine.

✳DO try seasoning with herbs or spices instead of salt; and avoid prepared foods high in sodium, such as many frozen dinners.

✳DON'T use whole milk, cream products, butter, or lard.

✳DON'T eat fried foods.

✳DON'T eat poultry skin (pull off *before* cooking).

✳DON'T use salad dressings (except for lowcal or yogurt), and don't allow restaurants to put dressings on your salad, or butter on your pancakes. Control these toppings yourself.

NUTRITION AND PERSONALITY TYPES

An important personality characteristic relating to nutrition, obesity, and health goals is called LOCUS OF CONTROL — meaning the source of the control in your life. People who believe that they control their own destinies ("internals") are said to have an *internal* locus of control, while those who believe that their destinies are in the hands of luck, fate, other people, society, or the world in general ("externals") have an *external* locus of control. Obviously, the person with an "internal locus of control" is better able to achieve long-term health goals.

The "internals" say to themselves that they can improve their health by choosing to follow a high-carbohydrate, low-fat nutritional plan. The "externals" say that they are too busy; social gatherings tempt them too much; their jobs require them to entertain and eat rich foods; mom always said, "Clean your plate;" stores show the wrong foods; restaurants just don't serve the right foods. And, of course, the weather is always too cold or too hot or too drizzly to go outside and exercise. And inside, there isn't enough room.

It is the externals who are more likely to abandon their health goals because they are long accus-

49

tomed to blaming others for their failures. Look deeply, honestly to see if you have "external" tendencies. Once having admitted it, you can set about CHANGING your view of life, and accepting responsibility for your future. You can begin to believe that you have the power to overcome such obstacles, and to control many aspects of your life — including your nutritional present and your healthful future.

8 RULES FOR EATING

To wrap up this chapter, we want to present you with some rules for eating which are quite easy to keep in mind.

They do not involve calorie counting or even avoidance of particular foods. They are based on extensive research and have been demonstrated to be effective for those who wish to take off weight.

Although we do not concentrate on weight loss to put you on the road to healthy living, the reduction occurs as a result of eating proper foods and getting regular exercise. The rules listed below are designed so that they do not deprive you of anything. They just ask you to pay attention to what you are doing.

Know What You Are Eating

The first four rules relate to what you do while you are eating.

Whenever you eat something:

RULE 1. Make sure you are seated, and preferably at a table. This means no eating while standing, walking, or even driving.

RULE 2. Don't do anything else. Don't read, watch TV, do a crossword puzzle, write a letter — nothing. Enjoy the food. Realize that you are eating it. Savor it.

RULE 3. Swallow what is in your mouth before you add more. And chew thoroughly what is in your mouth before you swallow. This also adds to your enjoyment of the food.

RULE 4. Talk only when your mouth is empty.

You may be violating all of these rules every day. If so, you probably can't totally change your behavior overnight. If you have a tendency to eat on the run, over the sink, as you drive to work, etc., concentrate on Rule #1 until you change your behavior and follow Rule #1 almost all of the time. That's what this is — behavior change — and you are the only one who can do it.

The remaining rules have to do with what psychologists call *stimulus control*. Many people with weight problems are extra-sensitive to external stimuli, such as the smell of freshly-baked cookies (the "externals" we just talked about). The smell is the stimulus. They smell them, they want them. The smell creates the desire or intensifies the desire.

If the smell of cookies has this effect on you, that is, causes you to buy or eat cookies, and you can't resist, then change your route. Don't go past that bakery or store. Choose another road.

To limit the effect of environmental stimuli on eating behavior:

RULE 5. Avoid those places that would cause you to eat extra (and unnecessary) food, such as bakeries or candy stores.

RULE 6. Don't shop for food when you are hungry.

RULE 7. Don't buy fattening foods, and get rid of any *now* in your house. If they are there (stimulus), you will eat them (response).

RULES 8 to 10 or 8 to 100. These are the rules you will make for yourself because you know what turns you on. Remember, you have five senses, and the sight, smell, sound (food cooking, pots and pans clanging, TV commercials), touch (keep your hands off the peanuts), or taste (can you eat just one potato chip? NO!) of food are ever present; are abundantly available.

Isolate these stimuli; get them out of your life. Let someone else make the Christmas candy and cook the birthday cakes. You can do the decorating.

The goal is to eliminate temptation and to stop being controlled by external stimuli. After you have practiced these rules, you will discover that you are consistently gaining more control over the things you do. You are moving from being an externally-controlled person to becoming internally-controlled. External factors can gang up on you. And external factors actually cause changes in your physiology. In one study, people who had not eaten for 18 hours were presented with a large juicy sizzling steak, filling the room with a delicious aroma. The hungry ones looked and smelled and thought, but before they started eating, blood samples were taken. Blood insulin levels rose in all of them and this was accompanied by greater feelings of hunger. The "externally controlled" members of the group showed greater increases in insulin production and in hunger than did the "internally controlled." So it isn't just a psychological desire, it becomes a physiological one as well.

Do you snack while you are talking on the phone? Remember RULE 2: don't let the phone control you. Eat when *you* decide, not when the phone rings or the TV commercial comes on.

Your goal is to be better, not perfect. And you get better step by step. As you keep improving and gaining control, you will be amazed at how good you feel.

CHAPTER 3

FAD DIET MYTHS AND DANGERS

"I'd better not eat that; I'm on a diet," is echoed millions of times each day, at ladies' luncheons, in factories, schools, corporate offices, and at the family dinner table. We (not just women) are a planet of dieters.

Millions of people around the world are now on a diet, just off a diet, or about to begin a diet. Many of these have already tried numerous diets, only to fail miserably, or succeed temporarily and then regain the weight lost, plus a few additional pounds for interest! Why does this happen? Are some types of diets unhealthy? Is weight reduction hopeless? What are the dangers of diets, and particularly of "FAD DIETS"?

What if you were not happy with a weight loss of only 1-2 pounds per week based on a calorie intake of 1,000 to 1,500 calories a day? You want to lose weight more quickly, so you cut back to 650 calories a day, by minimizing your carbohydrate calories. In that case, you run the same risks as one impatient dieter, John Thompson (not his real name).

John carried 225 pounds on a 5'9" frame. In January, he began the diet-and-exercise strategy in this book. In the first six months, he lost 14 pounds and three inches from his waist, but he was still not pleased with his progress. He wanted to reach 165 pounds more quickly.

John abandoned our program to follow one of the many high protein, high fat, low carbohydrate diets that have been touted in many diet books. During the next 12 weeks, he lost 40 pounds, and then weighed 171. However, during that time his energy level dropped due to the lack of complex carbohydrates, so he abandoned the exercise part of his program. Happy with his 171 pounds, he also abandoned his diet. In the next eight weeks, he regained the 40 pounds he lost on the "crash diet," plus the original 14 pounds lost on our program of proper nutrition combined with moderate exercise.

John Thompson's Vital Statistics in 1991-1992

Date	Weight	Waist in Inches	%Body Fat	Cholesterol Level	Triglycerides
Table 3-A					
Jan. 1991	225	45	35	274	235
June 1991	211	42	28	231	158
(John abandoned our program.)					
Sept. 1991	171	40	31	285	247
(John ended his fad diet)					
Nov. 1991	225	47	40	298	255

You might think that John was no worse off than when he started his diet almost a year ago. However, Table 3-A shows that this is not the case.

John's cholesterol has soared because of his high protein, high fat, low carbohydrate diet, and he is now at greater risk than ever for heart disease and other problems. This chart emphasizes the importance of following a program that can become a new *lifestyle*. Remember — health involves many factors, not just pounds, so health-conscious individuals should not be slaves to the scale.

FAD DIETS: FROM FRUSTRATION AND FAILURE TO DANGER

Most of these fad diets have one thing in common — they offer an eating program which severely limits calories, and may be deficient in basic vitamins and minerals.

A big reason most fad diets don't work is that much of the initial weight lost is water weight rather than fat, so they appear to be working if you focus only on the bathroom scale. But that fluid must eventually be replaced, for your health's sake, and when this occurs, your weight returns.

The extremely low caloric intake associated with these diets can also dangerously alter your metabolism. If the calorie total is too low, you may experience dehydration, fatigue, and bowel problems, and that's just the beginning. The human body is a machine programmed for survival. If the fuel is insufficient, your metabolism will shift to a starvation mode, becoming slower and slower, thus making it harder to lose weight because you will not be burning calories. And since your body is not receiving enough fuel for its metabolic engine, it must find fuel elsewhere — such as your existing muscle. So much of the weight loss will be from fluid and muscle. This will have a negative impact upon your fat-to-muscle ratio, your energy level, and your appearance. It can even damage your major organs.

In addition to the physical risks, there are emotional ones. Fad diets tend to be frustrating and difficult to follow, which leads to high failure rates, depression, moodiness, then more failure and deeper depression.

Even after you stop dieting, your metabolism will continue in its starvation mode for a period of time. Your metabolic rate will be low because you lost much of the muscle tissue that had raised your metabolic rate and burned calories. As you begin to eat "normally," with a body (and mind) still operating in a starvation mode, you regain all of the lost weight, plus additional pounds the body thinks it needs to protect itself against future starvation.

Avoid all fad diets — including any diet which promises rapid weight loss of more than 2 pounds per week. It probably took years for you to acquire your body fat. You can't expect to lose it in a few weeks!

8 MYTHS ASSOCIATED WITH DIETING

Dieters are often their own worst enemies, because they have so many misconceptions about diet and health. These myths come from fad-diet books, celebrity testimonials, and misinformation from well-meaning friends and family.

MYTH 1. SKIPPING MEALS WILL HELP YOU LOSE WEIGHT

Overweight people are often meal skippers, and the meal they are most likely to skip is breakfast — the metabolically most important meal of the day. But skipping meals leads to weight gain rather than weight loss, for several reasons:

First, when you skip meals, particularly break-fast, your metabolic rate decreases, because after a long night with no food, your body doesn't know when it's going to be fed again, so it slows down and conserves energy. Without breakfast, the body never gets the fuel to raise the metabolic rate.

According to a study at George Washington University, *people who eat breakfast have a metabolic rate 4-5 percent higher* than those who skip breakfast. In one experiment, those who ate only in the morning were able to lose weight, even when they took in a whopping 2000 calories. (The usual caloric intake for an entire day when "dieting" is about 1000, 1500 tops!) Those who skipped breakfast and ate 2000 calories in the afternoon, actually gained weight, because the *calories are used differently by the body throughout the day*, depending on the balance of two hormones — insulin and glucagon.

What? You say you get sick if you eat breakfast? That's only because your body is not used to it. We recommend you begin a *gradual* change — begin your day with a bagel and crushed fruit (no butter or cream cheese). It will take a few weeks for your body to adjust so you can eat foods listed in the Breakfast chart, Table 2-B. Breakfast will help fuel your furnace (metabolic rate) for better health and weight loss.

Second, when you skip a meal you are likely to eat the wrong foods at your next meal, and take larger portions to unconsciously "catch up." Meal skippers are also more likely to snack or gorge on unhealthy, high-fat foods between meals. Finally, meal skippers will have less energy, will tend to live a sedentary existence, missing out on most forms of heart-stimulating activity.

MYTH 2. THE FASTER I LOSE THE WEIGHT, THE BETTER OFF I AM

Patience is in such short supply in the Western world, particularly with weight reduction. Most people want to accomplish their goals in the best and fastest way. But these terms are mutually exclusive. For taking off weight and keeping it off, rapid weight loss is a poor strategy, because, like meal-skipping, these pounds are lost mostly through muscle and fluid. This lowers the metabolic rate and energy level, making it harder to burn calories through exercise, and depends on an eating strategy which cannot be followed on a long-term basis.

MYTH 3. ALL CALORIES AFFECT YOUR BODY IN THE SAME WAY

The truth is that the *source* of your calories is more important than the total number of calories. Remember this when you shop, when you put fork to mouth — one gram of fat contains nine calories, while one gram of carbohydrate contains only four calories.

Unlike fat calories, those from complex carbohydrates increase your metabolic rate, giving you the energy to carry out your exercise program, and giving your body the energy to burn fat. Second, research shows that *fat calories are more easily converted to body fat than are carbohydrate calories.* This evidence supports what has always seemed obvious: your body responds differently to carrots than to chocolate cheesecake!

A bonus is that on a complex carbohydrate diet you may eat more than you thought, while maintaining or even decreasing your weight, and improving your fat-to-muscle ratio. However, you must COMMIT yourself to just say "no" to those high-fat foods which seem to beat a path to your hips and abdomen.

MYTH 4. POUNDS LOST IS THE BEST INDEX OF THE SUCCESS OF A DIET

The best index of the type of weight you are losing is the fit of your clothes. If they are becoming loose, you are probably losing fat. But, if you've lost mostly muscle and water, your clothes will quickly become snug again as the weight returns in the form of fat rather than muscle. Remember that your key goal is to constantly improve your fat-to-muscle ratio.

MYTH 5. DIET PILLS ARE THE DIETER'S BEST FRIEND

Over-the-counter diet pills artificially speed up and stimulate your body, and/or have a diuretic effect and decrease the fluid in your body. This does cause you to lose weight, but only in the short run. The weight returns as soon as fluids are naturally replenished when you stop taking the pills. You have not lost the body fat, nor naturally speeded up your metabolic rate, nor improved your fat-to-muscle ratio.

MYTH 6. POTATOES, BREADS, AND PASTA SHOULD BE AVOIDED DURING A DIET

Actually, these foods are rich in complex carbohydrates and should play an important role in your caloric intake. If your diet tells you to eliminate them, consider a different diet. The problem is not with the foods but with what you add to them — potatoes smothered with sour cream, bread slathered with butter, pasta served with mounds of meat sauce. Learn to enjoy these healthy foods in their natural *naked* form, or with healthier, leaner toppings — low fat yogurt on a baked potato, or a meatless and creamless sauce on pasta, a little crushed fruit as a jam on bread. Or try a delicious baked potato *au naturel*, pasta with a little garlic and olive oil *all ' italiana*, or unadorned good-as-cake whole grain bread. This alternative can be savored on a permanent basis. The more you eat them, the more you like them. And they certainly like you.

MYTH 7. DIETS REQUIRE "SPECIAL FOODS "

Some diet programs today provide people with expensive, and yes, in many cases, healthy foods in prepackaged, correct-sized portions. But proper diet food is simply low-fat, healthy food from the six basic food groups, and need cost no more than high-fat, unhealthy foods. In fact, the most expensive foods are those highest in fat calories — cakes, steaks, and cheeses!

MYTH 8. DIETS CAN'T WORK FOR ME — EVERYONE IN MY FAMILY IS FAT

The role of heredity cannot be denied. It isn't fair, but a person with a family history of obesity simply has to work harder to control weight. If you have a history of obesity in your family, it is particularly important for the sake of your heart to follow a healthy lifestyle. Many conditions passed down from our ancestors are not under our control. Obesity is!

THE YO-YO EFFECT: WHY DIETERS REGAIN THEIR LOST WEIGHT

More diet books are sold than books on any other self-help topic. This is true because more than 90% of all dieters fail, and think the answer is another diet book. So they lose weight quickly on one diet, but gain it back—plus a few extra pounds, then on to a new diet, and their weight goes down again, then up, then a new diet, and on and on. This cycle is called the "YO-YO EFFECT," and most diet programs contribute to the yo-yo effect in a number of ways:

1. Extreme restriction of calories slows down the metabolism, which leads to a smaller weight loss each week, which leads to your abandoning the diet.

2. Complicated, confusing, time-consuming regimens make dieters abandon them in frustration.

3. Failing to emphasize the importance of exercise makes the dieter more likely to regain lost weight.

4. Limiting dieters to one or a few foods makes it difficult for these programs to be sustained — psychologically or physically. You can't be expected to eat only grapefruit for the rest of your life.

5.Recommending high fat intake (like a steak a day), results in short-term weight loss but actually increases the percentage of body fat, and cholesterol level.

6.Decreasing bodily fluids either by dietary limitations or diuretics is only temporary. When your body replenishes the lost fluids, your weight returns.

Think what the repeated changes of the yo-yo effect do to your heart, your other organs, and your morale. But the yo-yo effect cannot be blamed solely on the diets — the attitudes of dieters themselves also contribute to it, if they:

1. plan on losing weight very rapidly;

2. plan on returning to their old eating habits after losing the desired amount of weight;

3. refuse to exercise;

4. unconsciously expect to regain the lost weight, because they failed at previous diets;

5. skip meals;

6. blame their obesity on external, uncontrollable factors... such as genetics or having to cook for the family, or the need to entertain lavishly;

7. hate their weight loss program, the foods they feel forced to eat, or the loss of "favorite" foods.

Pick a diet which is a non-diet, which is a lifestyle. Pick foods that are healthy, that you can love for a lifetime. The critical word here is PATIENCE. *Weight is not gained overnight nor can it be lost overnight.*

THE DANGERS OF FASTING

Many people claim that the only way they have lost weight is through a total or modified fast. While medically supervised fasts have unfortunately become popular, the most dangerous fasts are self-imposed. If these self-designed programs are continued for a long period of time, damage to your mind and body, even death, can result.

When you fast, you can expect initially to lose a significant amount of weight. But soon your metabolic rate decreases along with your ability to burn fat. Much of the weight lost on a fast is fluid and muscle fiber. This can leave you fatigued, dehydrated, suffering vertigo, even hallucinations. Longer-term fasts can damage your respiratory system and kidneys, may lead to a wide range of other medical problems, and also cause serious emotional problems such as depression.

If a fast is continued for a long time, your body will burn skeletal muscle and finally even the heart muscle for fuel, causing irreversible damage to that organ. People who suffer from anorexia nervosa, in which a modified fast may persist for years, are at especially high risk of such problems.

One of the saddest truths is that many people who fast, particularly women, are really only five or ten pounds beyond some aesthetic ideal which generally bears little or no relationship to the reality of an attractive and healthy body. Women should accept themselves as something other than a Barbie-doll size five.

ANALYSIS OF FAD DIET PROGRAMS

One of the most important ways you can protect your long-term health is by steering clear of dangerous fad diets. While it is not feasible to discuss each of the dozens of well-known diets, it is possible to describe the general types. The good news is that there are many healthy programs. But as a consumer, you must learn to recognize which ones are healthy, and for whom they are appropriate.

LIQUID DIETS

In the 1970's, a number of people actually died from liquid protein diets, because these diets lacked many essential nutrients. *Optifast*®, (manufactured by Sandoz Nutrition, Corp.), the diet Oprah Winfrey made famous, is today's most popular totally liquid diet, and is vastly superior to the liquid diets of the 1970's. It provides proper nutrients within an extremely low calorie base, and is legitimately offered only through medical facilities, and only to people at least 30%, or 50 pounds, above their proper weight. A key part of the *Optifast*® and similar programs is the ongoing monitoring by a health professional. The big problem is that, with any totally liquid diet, you are not practicing proper eating habits because you are not eating food. One final drawback is the expense — usually several thousand dollars. *Optifast*® has also declined in popularity since Oprah regained the 67lbs. she lost on the liquid diet.

Another popular, and heavily advertised liquid diet is the *Ultra Slim Fast* ® program (manufactured by Slim Fast Foods, Co.). This over-the-counter product is taken as your breakfast and lunch, along with a balanced light dinner. Assuming that you do indeed eat a balanced dinner, this program can be safe in the short run. However, you must face a basic reality — you cannot expect to limit yourself to one solid meal a day for the rest of your life.

OTHER EXTREMELY LOW CALORIE DIETS

These diets may be based on either liquids or solids. The most famous, the *Cambridge Diet*, is limited to approximately 330 calories per day. We do not believe that you can expect to consume all appropriate nutrients on only 300-400 calories per day. Most programs of this type are subject to all the dangers of fasting.

HIGH CARBOHYDRATE DIETS

These diets are an example of too much of a good thing. While we do recommend a diet high in complex carbohydrates, we also stress that 15-20% of your calories should come from meat and dairy protein, and 15-20% from fat sources. "Balance" means some from all the food categories. It is extremely unwise to limit yourself to grapefruit only or, as the *Beverly Hills Diet* suggests, six weeks of fruit only. This approach can lead to a variety of problems including diarrhea and hair loss, because your body rebels against such a one-sided diet.

LOW CARBOHYDRATE DIETS

These diets limit the individual to mostly fat and/or protein sources for calories. This can lead to short-term weight loss by depleting your body of necessary fluids (which come rushing right back along with the weight). This is not good for either your metabolism or your fat-to-muscle ratio. And obviously getting large amounts of your calories from fat sources can also raise your cholesterol level. Avoid diets which either ignore or severely limit foods from the carbohydrate group. All such high protein and high fat diets can be dangerous.

APPROVED DIETS

Diets which we recommend provide high levels of complex carbohydrates and modest amounts of fat and protein. Healthy diets, such as the *Weight Watcher's® Program*, allow for 15-20% of calories from fat and a minimum of 60% of calories from carbohydrates. These programs provide steady and reliable weight loss, and can be adhered to on a healthy long-term basis.

QUESTIONS TO ASK WHEN EVALUATING A PARTICULAR DIET

While it is always best to check with your family doctor, the following questions should be of some help to you. Ideally, the answer to each question should be *yes*.

1. Does the diet provide at least 1000 calories per day?

2. Does the diet limit fat to 20% or less of total calorie intake?

3. Does the diet include food from all six of the food groups: fruits; vegetables; grains (bread, cereal, rice, pasta); dairy; meat, poultry, fish; and oils)?

4. Does the diet provide 60-65% of the calories from complex carbohydrates (fruits, vegetables, whole grain products)?

5. Does the diet provide daily protein sources?

6. Is the diet based on slow and steady weight loss?

7. Does the diet provide three or more meals per day?

8. Does the diet encourage drinking plenty of water (6-8 glasses per dy to cleanse the body of toxins), and other fluids, such as juices and herbal teas?

9. Does it avoid diet pills?

10. Does the diet include or support an exercise regimen?

11. Is the diet based on hard evidence rather than on testimonials?

12. Do the authors of the diet have reasonable credentials?

13. Is the diet supported by scientific evidence?
14. Is the diet safe?
15. Is the diet practical?
16. Is the diet affordable?
17. Is the diet likely to help you meet your personal goals?
18. Is the diet based upon principles which you can live with for the rest of your life?

If you have answered "no" to several of these questions, we strongly suggest that you have the diet checked by a family physician or other health professional prior to undertaking it.

CHAPTER 4

FUNdamentals OF EXERCISE — FOR BODY, HEART, AND MIND

Unfortunately, most of the people who constantly badger you to exercise — doctors, friends, Aunt Sally — either don't know or fail to tell you why you should. Even many doctors fail to explain the nature and benefits of a good exercise program. This chapter will try to help you establish a regimen you can make as a part of your new lifestyle, leading toward a longer, healthier, more joyful LIFE.

EXERCISE! EXERCISE!! EXERCISE!!! The body ages faster when it is not exercised. People who exercise look and feel years younger. Ever notice that glow of youth about older people who regularly work out? They look as though they're on top of the world, because they are on top of their health.

When athletes are forced to take bed rest for as little as three weeks, they lose 30 percent of their former level of fitness. Think about that the next time you plant your non-athletic body in front of the "tube."

If there is one clear lesson in diet and health, it is that a successful weight-loss strategy must include aerobic exercise, if you are to reach and maintain your ideal weight and fitness.

If you're willing to take the plunge on cutting the calories, then go the whole nine yards and start moving that body. Jog, bike, skate, ski, swim, hike, jump rope, do fast walking, run after the dog — get your face flushed, your heart pounding, your lungs expanding. That's what burns the fat off. Of course, individuals on fad diets or self-imposed fasts never have the energy to get up and go, but if you are following a reasonable dietary program you will have the energy, and exercise is the best way to decrease your fat and increase your muscle.

Anyone can exercise. People in wheel chairs put themselves through the New York Marathon, or play basketball — just to prove they can do it. All it takes is WILL.

BEGINNING: THE FIRST STEP IS THE HARDEST

Jill has decided to begin an exercise program. She rummages through the attic for the old gym sneakers she wore 20 years ago. As soon as she finds the sneakers, she begins her program — with a ten mile jog. Result:

1. Exhaustion
2. Failure
3. Disgust
4. Orthopedic injury (knee, ankle, etc.)
5. Respiratory or cardiovascular difficulties
6. Returns the sneakers to the attic for another 20 years

How should you prepare effectively for an exercise program? That depends on your age, the type of program, the date of your last physical, your current medical condition, your family history — and basic health indices such as blood pressure and cholesterol level.

So the first step for most people is a visit to a doctor for clearance to begin. This is especially important if any of the following conditions apply:

1. Sedentary and over 35 years of age
2. Have not exercised regularly during the last five years
3. Overweight
4. Smokes
5. Known health problems
6. Family history of cardiovascular disease
7. Have not had a physical exam during the last two years
8. Planning an overly ambitious, vigorous program

Even if you do not fit any of the above categories, you should have professional advice to find the best type of program for your particular needs. It is a good idea to supplement the information in this book with a visit to your physician, and also an athletic trainer at a health (spa) center, a sports medicine center, or the "Y."

Let's assume your doctor says it's okay to begin an exercise program. Which exercises should you choose? It's best to start with stretching, then brisk walking. Walking is great exercise because it gives you the benefits of more strenuous forms but few of the risks. And it's "free" exercise. A sample walking-and-stretching program is presented later in this chapter.

Your footwear must be tailored to the type of exercise. Many injuries from jogging, and even walking, are caused by improper footwear. Today footwear is exercise specific. Because of different kinds of stress on the foot and ankle, different types of shoes must be used by walkers, joggers, and basketball players. For your first pair, we recommend you discuss your needs with the trained personnel at a store specializing in athletic footwear. Be prepared to pay at least fifty dollars for quality shoes. You're looking for trouble if you begin a vigorous walking program with a ten-dollar pair of sneakers.

TWO TYPES OF EXERCISE: AEROBIC AND ANAEROBIC

AEROBIC exercise is *continuous* activity over a significant period of time which involves large muscle groups. It results in an increased heart rate and an overall increase in the demand on your cardiovascular system. That means heavy perspiring, heart-thumping, hard-breathing sustained exercise. It stimulates your circulation, and cleans out the stale air. *Aerobic* exercise, including aerobic classes, can be high impact or low impact.

HIGH IMPACT is the kind you see when people are jumping around in the gym, as well as jogging, jumping rope, doing jumping jacks, or down-hill skiing. The term "high impact" means that you are pounding approximately four times your body weight into the ground. If you are a 150-pound runner you may be supporting 600 pounds on the *front part* of one foot, and then the other foot, or one foot at a time, thousands of times daily. No wonder runners and joggers get shin splints.

LOW IMPACT exercise, like walking, always keeps one foot squarely on the ground, in a heel-toe movement. Walking builds the shins and knees, rather than tearing them down, as running or jogging can do. Other low-impact exercises are bike riding, cross-country skiing, rowing, using a Nordic Track® machine, hiking, mountain biking, and that most perfect of all body workouts, swimming.

ANAEROBIC exercise involves more intense activity in relatively brief bursts which does *not* raise the heart rate for an extended period of time. Examples are sprinting for less than three minutes, or playing sports such as football, even ice hockey. These require tremendous bursts of energy followed by slow-or-no action.

Another anaerobic exercise is WEIGHT-LIFT-ING, which also requires short bursts of energy. Weight-lifting strengthens the bones and tones the muscles. Lifting weights is of tremendous benefit to older adults, making their bones more dense made porous by osteoporosis. Weight-lifting is now considered essential for an older person recovering from a broken bone. The shocking truth is that 50% of women over 60 can't lift 10 pounds, but one study indicated that eighty, even ninety-year-olds can triple their muscle strength with as little as 8-9 weeks of training.

A note of caution: Health problems such as heart disease can make certain anaerobic movements dangerous because they cause brief but substantial increases in blood pressure. So always consult a physician and a trainer before beginning a weight-training program.

We're frequently asked about organized sports. Many people claim they are in terrific shape because they bowl, golf, play softball, or tennis. All these offer benefits of relaxation plus calorie burning, but lack one or more of the basic components of aerobic exercise. In softball, most of your time is spent sitting on the bench or standing in the field, with occasional bursts of anaerobic exercise in the form of chasing fly balls and running bases. Bowling requires four or five slow steps, 10-20 times per game. Tennis is an energetic game, especially singles, but its aerobic value is limited by the time spent standing, awaiting serves, retrieving balls, and changing courts. Golf is mildly beneficial as long as you don't ride around in a cart.

Enjoy these sports as a *supplement* to your aerobic program, not as a substitute for it. They can't take the place of brisk walking, jogging, swimming, cycling, or rowing. *Get in shape to play your sport. Don't play a sport to get in shape.*

10 MYTHS ABOUT EXERCISE

There are many myths used to rationalize an unwillingness to get up and make your body move. Here are some which might be holding you back.

MYTH 1. THE JIM FIXX MYTH - EXERCISE KILLS

Contrary to rumor, Jim Fixx, the renowned runner, did not die from a heart attack caused by running. Fixx had a very poor genetic history. His father died of a heart attack at age 43. Other males in the family also succumbed to heart disease at very young ages. In addition, Fixx was a smoker, with a very high cholesterol level at the time of his death. In reality, he probably survived to his ripe old age of 52 because of his running. Given a different family history, Jim Fixx would probably be running for decades more.

MYTH 2. NO PAIN - NO GAIN

True, some discomfort may have to be endured to become a world-class athlete. But there is nothing painful in the level of aerobic exercise needed to improve your health and overall fitness. Vigorous walking is not painful, it's exhilarating. The important thing is to find a level that is beneficial for you. If you over train, you actually decrease your performance level. Young female athletes and aerobic instructors who over train may actually stop menstruating, or develop stress fractures and even a youthful form of osteoporosis.

MYTH 3. MANY PEOPLE GET ENOUGH EXERCISE ON THE JOB

Even on an active job, it is unlikely that you participate in 30 or more continuous minutes of aerobic activity (unless you are an aerobic instructor). Hard work and perspiration do not necessarily improve aerobic fitness. Workers such as roofers and builders still need an exercise program.

MYTH 4. EXERCISE INCREASES YOUR APPETITE

In fact, the opposite is true. Aerobic exercise actually *decreases* your appetite — it certainly takes your mind off food. But, do be careful to drink plenty of fluids before and after an aerobic workout. If, in the short run, you lose water weight, you will feel fatigued, with a decreased metabolic rate — which will cause you, in the long run, to lose less weight.

MYTH 5. EXERCISE LEAVES YOU FEELING FATIGUED AND SORE

This won't happen if you exercise at the right level for you. To avoid *post-exercise fatigue* and sore-ness, follow these simple guidelines:

a. Stretch — before you exercise as a warm-up, and afterwards as a cool-down.

b. Observe the hard-easy principle — follow a day of hard exercise with a day of easy exercise.

c. Cross-train by alternating your activities. If you ride a stationary bicycle on Monday, walk on Tuesday.

d. Take one or two days off per week.

MYTH 6. EXERCISE IS FOR THE YOUNG

Professional football or basketball is for young people, but older adults can walk, swim, cycle, ski, jog, or row, at their appropriate levels. There are eighty-year-olds who finish marathons, ninety-year-olds who cross-country ski, and many oldsters who swim 20-30 laps each day. Even if you have not exercised in fifty years, it is not too late to start — it is too late NOT to start!

MYTH 7. YOU ARE TOO OUT OF SHAPE TO BEGIN AN EXERCISE PROGRAM

You may be too out of shape to begin a *vigorous* exercise program, but physicians not only permit but encourage the vast majority of their patients to become involved in an aerobic regimen. Just start slowly and increase gradually as your fitness improves.

MYTH 8. EXERCISE ENABLES YOU TO EAT ANYTHING YOU WANT

That's almost true. Since exercise burns calories and increases your metabolic rate to burn more calories — it certainly does allow you one "FUN" a day, be it a glass of wine, a piece of cake, or an ice cream cone — we do not live by VEG alone. But no amount of exercise can compensate for the harm you do your body by a consistent pattern of eating high-cholesterol, high-fat foods.

MYTH 9. EXERCISE PROGRAMS ARE EXPENSIVE

While you may not have the funds to join a trendy spa, you can probably afford a pair of good walking shoes.

MYTH 10. EXERCISE IS BORING

Exercise is boring only if you allow it to be. If walking is your sport, you can avoid boredom by going with a friend, listening to music, changing your route, counting red cars, playing mental gymnastics like trying to name state capitals or all the players on your favorite baseball team. Or do interval training by varying your walking pace — walk two minutes at 125 steps per minute, then one minute at 135 steps per minute — long steps then baby steps (wear your sports watch). Whatever games you get into, enjoy your walk. That's the whole point of "working" towards wellness — the enjoyment of LIFE.

BODY BENEFITS OF AEROBIC EXERCISE

When you walk, cycle, swim, hike, ski, or jog, your heart rate increases as the demands on it increase. And with each beat the heart pumps more blood and becomes stronger because, like all muscles, it strengthens with exercise. Your heart may actually become larger (a healthy change) in the course of a long-term program. (This is not to be confused with enlargement of the heart, commonly present in heart disease.) Your arteries will dilate to permit the increased blood flow. Some people even develop extra blood vessels, which can redirect the flow of blood in critical situations such as a heart attack, minimizing the damage. And, of course, your body will burn more fat calories as you build muscle.

Physical and mental benefits of an aerobic exercise program are almost endless. Some are:
1. Increased energy
2. Lower blood pressure
3. Higher levels of HDL (good cholesterol)
4. Lower levels of triglycerides
5. Fewer injuries while performing everyday activities (because your body is more in tune with itself)
6. Weight reduction
7. DECREASED APPETITE
8. Increased metabolic rate
9. Lower risk of heart disease
10. Decreased resting heart rate
11. Lower risk of some forms of cancer
12. Increased ability to handle stress

13. Decreased anxiety
14. Decreased need to rely on drugs or alcohol as relaxants
15. Fewer common illnesses
16. Decreased risk of osteoporosis
17. Fewer back strains
18. Better outlook on life
19. Better quality of life
20. Higher self-esteem
21. Meeting healthier, more interesting people
22. LONGER LIFE

These benefits should be enough to motivate anyone. Perhaps the best advice we can give you is to talk to people who have been in an aerobic exercise program for several years. They will verify the benefits we've discussed, and will probably add a few of their own.

EXERCISE QUIZ

Are you getting enough exercise in your battle for wellness in mind and body? Evaluate your program by answering these three questions. Your score is determined by multiplying all three of the point-scores. (For example, if you score 5 points on each question, your total score would be 5 x 5 x 5, or 125 — the maximum possible score.)

1. How frequently do you exercise?
   a. 6 times per week (5 points)
   b. 4-5 times per week (4 points)
   c. 3 times per week (3 points)
   d. 1-2 times per week (2 points)
   e. 1-2 times per month (1 point)

IF YOU DON'T EXERCISE AT ALL (0 POINTS) STOP HERE. DON'T BOTHER ANSWERING QUESTIONS 2 & 3 – YOUR SCORE IS ZERO!

2. How would you describe your exercise program?
   a. Frequent heavy sweating (5 points)
   b. Frequent light sweating (4 points)
   c. Occasional light sweating (3 points)
   d. Mild exercise below Target Heart Rate as described in the next chapter (2 points)
   e. Slow walking as if window-shopping (1 point)

3. How long is your average workout, excluding warm-up and cool-down?
   a. 45 minutes or more (5 points)
   b. 30 minutes (4 points)
   c. 20 minutes (3 points)

d. 15 minutes (2 points)
e. 10 minutes or less (1 point)

80-125 EXCELLENT. Your exercise program is an optimal one which should contribute greatly to your wellness.

60-79 VERY GOOD. You have a solid program. At most, it could use some fine tuning. Keep up the good work.

40-59 GOOD. You're doing better than most people, but there is room for improvement. Consider increasing the frequency, intensity, and/or duration of your workouts.

20-39 FAIR. You are moderately active, but you must upgrade your exercise program if it is to contribute to your health in a positive way.

0-19 POOR. You are doing very little and need to get involved in some vigorous activity. Today is the best day to take the steps needed to become an active exerciser. Get up and get going now and loosen up — start with the stretches described in the next chapter under "Warm-up."

CHAPTER 5

BASIC SECRETS OF A GOOD EXERCISE PROGRAM

A good program must work in both the short and long term. You need a LONG-TERM plan of weekly and monthly regimens so that you will avoid too much, as well as too little, exercise. In your SHORT-TERM PLAN of almost-daily exercise, the three basic components are the WARM-UP, the AEROBIC EXERCISE, and the COOL-DOWN.

WARM-UP

The general purpose here is to prepare the body. This involves the muscles and joints as well as the cardiovascular system. If you skip this step, you may injure yourself or experience other discomfort. The warm-up should begin with some gentle relaxation in the form of slow lazy movements, including walking, followed by stretching exercises, which ideally, should stretch all key parts of the body:

QUADRICEPS — These are the muscles in the front of the thigh. The quads can easily be stretched by standing close to a wall, chair, or tree. While facing it, place your left hand on the wall or tree, for balance, and slowly bend your right leg backward.

Put your right hand around your right ankle and pull your heel toward your buttocks. Hold this stretch for 10 seconds — relax your leg, then repeat two more times. Now do exactly the same thing three times with the other leg. Try *not* to bounce or jerk while stretching. We now know that *bouncing can cause injury to muscles, ligaments, even to joints.*

HAMSTRINGS — These are the muscles in the back of the thigh which run from the buttocks to the area above and behind the knee. The hamstrings can be stretched by sitting on the floor.

To stretch the right hamstrings, sit with your right leg out straight in front of you with the toes pointed upward towards the ceiling, keeping that knee as close to the floor as possible, slightly bent if necessary.

Now with your left knee bent to the outside, place your left sole against the inside of your right thigh just above the knee, in a figure-four position. Lean forward, keeping your right leg as straight as possible, and r-e-a-c-h as far as you can (without pain) with both hands toward your right foot or ankle.

You can feel the stretch in the back of your right thigh and up your back. Hold for 10 seconds, then relax by sitting upright. Repeat two more times. Reverse the process for your left hamstrings (three times as before). This is a splendid exercise for your back as well.

CALF MUSCLES AND ANKLES — Stand two to three feet from a solid surface such as a wall or tree, and place your hands against the wall. To stretch the right calf and ankle, stretch your right leg behind you, keeping both legs straight. Now slowly bend the left leg forward, keeping both heels flat on the ground. Lean toward the wall and you will feel the stretch. Hold for 10 seconds; repeat two more times. Reverse the process for the left leg.

IMPORTANT NOTE: Balancing both sides is extremely important in stretching. If you stretch one leg or arm three times for 10 seconds, you must do exactly this in the same way for the other leg or arm. Otherwise you could end up with lopsided muscles. Honest!

BACK — Lower back pain strikes most adults in our sedentary society. To relieve this pain we recommend three different back stretches — for exercisers and non-exercisers alike.

The first stretch requires you to lie on your back with both knees bent. Then use your hands to pull your bent right leg up to your chest and hold for ten seconds. Do this three times, and then repeat for the left leg.

For the second exercise, perform the same movement as above, except with both legs at the same time. Again repeat this stretch three times.

The third stretch is perhaps the most important. Lay on your back, feet flat on the floor, knees bent, hands behind your head. Cross your right ankle over your left leg, and rest it on your left thigh just above the knee. With shoulders flat, lower your right knee to the right until it touches the ground or comes as close to it as you are able. Hold for ten seconds. Do three times, and then reverse the process for the left leg. This helps to prevent lower back strains from quickly twisting the body to pick up an object, or catch something from falling.

THE AEROBIC PHASE

You are now ready to begin. Your basic goals in aerobic exercising are cardiovascular conditioning, weight and fat loss, stress reduction, lowering of cholesterol and blood pressure, as well as strengthening your bones and toning your muscles.

To help you remember the key elements of a successful aerobic exercise program, we have formed a "code word" for you, from the letters *F.I.T.*, for *Frequency, Intensity, and Time.*

F IS FOR FREQUENCY. A good aerobic program includes at least *three* sessions a week, and increases gradually to 4 or 5 sessions (absolute tops,

6). When you get up to 5 per week, use cross-training by alternating your activities — walk briskly on Monday, bike or swim on Tuesday. This prevents boredom, and exercises different muscles. Also, follow the hard-easy principle — one day hard, next day easy. Pushing yourself without a break, and not cross-training increases the danger of injury or drop out.

I IS FOR INTENSITY. Your workout should raise your heart rate to within the TARGET HEART RATE ZONE. The calculations for this are:

Maximal Heart Rate = 220 minus your age
(for a 40-year-old: 220 - 40 = 180)
Target Heart Rate = 60 to 85% of your maximal heart rate (See Table 5-A)

You can check your heart rate either on the side of your neck under the jaw or on the left wrist below the base of your thumb. Use your index and middle fingers to check the pulse — or buy a pulse meter that clips onto an ear lobe or finger or wear it as a watch. These can be bought for less than $40.

As you begin an exercise program, the heart rate should be checked frequently during a workout. If your heart rate is too slow, speed up your exercise. If

TARGET HEART RATE ZONE		
Age	Maximal Heart Rate	Target Heart Rate Zone
25	195	117-166
30	190	114-162
35	185	111-157
40	180	108-153
45	175	105-149
50	170	102-144
55	165	99-140
60	160	96-138
65	155	93-132

Table 5-A

it is too fast, slow down gradually until your heart rate falls within the target zone. As your physical condition improves, you can begin to perform more of your workout at a higher rate than the minimum 60% of your maximal heart rate.

T IS FOR TIME. An optimal workout includes a minimum of 30 minutes within the target heart rate zone. If you're currently out of shape or haven't worked out recently, you should slowly work your way up to the 30-minute mark.

The particular form of exercise is not important. Choose one that fits your interests, lifestyle, and current physical condition. If possible, exercise at the same time of day throughout the week. Your body and mind *adjust* better to a regular routine.

Making drastic changes in your exercise schedule can create problems similar to those of shift workers (those of you on afternoon or midnight shifts, must adjust your lifestyle, for when ever you wake up that is your breakfast time). Your body is simply more comfortable if it is kept on a consistent schedule. Consistency has the additional benefit of increasing your likelihood of doing the exercise. It prevents you from delaying and possible avoiding exercise.

Avoid exercising within 2 hours after eating — unless it's a very light meal. Exercise takes blood from the stomach to the limbs, hindering breakdown of food. And try not to exercise in extreme heat and humidity. If you must, then decrease the intensity and time by 10-15%. Or find a shopping mall to trot up and down in. You'll be surprised how many people are doing just that.

COOL-DOWN

This is extremely important but is often over-looked. Cool-down enables your heart rate to decrease gradually to its resting rate, and helps prevent post-exercise soreness and muscular tightness. Begin your cool-down with a brief 4-to-5 minute slow walk, followed by the stretching exercises described earlier. *Allow 40 to 50 minutes for the whole workout process – warm-up, aerobics, cool-down.*

You now have the basic ingredients of a sound exercise program. Keep the following tips in mind:

1. See your physician should you feel any significant discomfort while exercising.

2. Wear comfortable loose-fitting cotton clothing for summer workouts, layers of clothing for winter workouts.

3. Never exercise aerobically wearing a rubber suit (unless it's a sport which requires one).

4. Regularly replace your footwear.

5. Walk in pairs or groups, to increase your pleasure index, and to keep to your regimen.

6. Breathe deeply as you exercise.

7. Stand up straight while you walk.

8. Avoid exaggerated arm movements during your walk; they wear you out faster.

9. Drink plenty of water to replenish fluids lost through perspiration. If you wait until you thirst — you're down a quart of water!
10. Enjoy yourself.

EXERCISE AND THE OLDER ADULT

A middle-aged father we know was recently observed on a father-and-son trip. When the man learned that a one-mile walk was planned, he panicked. He convinced the group that he could never complete such an event — as if a one-mile walk were an Olympic event. His lack of fitness is affecting not only his quality of life but that of his son. One can only wonder what the future holds for this obese chain-smoking father.

But the good news is that it is never too late for him to start an exercise program, to stop smoking, or change his high-fat diet. Sunbonnet Sue, famous marathon runner, is in her eighties. She began running in her sixties — because she didn't like the way she was stiffening up from arthritis.

The average life-expectancy in the 1990's is 75, and there is no reason it should not go up to 85 in the future. As longevity increases we will need cooperation from the middle-aged and older adults (which includes all of us, sooner or later, if we are lucky) in lifestyle changes, if we are to realize our potential in longevity, much less enjoy those years when they come.

The most needed CHANGES are smoking cessation, improved diet, increased exercise, and decreased use of alcohol and other drugs — legal and illegal. Older adults must come to realize that retirement does not mean leading a sedentary life; it does not mean retiring from life.

Exercise can improve not only health and longevity, but the very quality of life. It gives zest, and enables one to return to activities associated with youth, to become more involved with other people, to enjoy time with children and grandchildren.

One concern among older adults, who may have spent decades sitting behind a desk, is that they might be risking broken bones or a heart attack when they begin to exercise. This need not be a fear, as long as your doctor evaluates your family history and your current physical condition, based on screening procedures such as a stress test, to detect any existing cardiovascular disease or other problems.

Once this has been done, choose the form(s) of exercise which you would most enjoy. Walking is an ideal first choice. As you will want to gradually increase the intensity, a sample program covering your first 12 weeks of walking is shown on the following page.

If you wish to exercise more than four days a week, you should "cross-train" — alternate your exercises to keep from getting stale. And remember not to do more than six days of exercise.

The weights, beginning in week 5, are optional. They increase your cardiovascular workout all the more, decrease that "tire" around your waist, flatten your belly, and for females, help to lift and separate!

Weights are held in the hands and swung in a natural motion as you stride along. Feel free to make up your own movements, to your own rhythm. In the beginning, keep it simple, and take it very easy. We don't want you to crack yourself on the head with a dumbbell.

Speed is much less important than consistency. Begin with a steady, undemanding pace. If you cannot converse comfortably, you are going too fast. If

WALKING PROGRAM FOR OLDER
OR
OUT-OF-SHAPE ADULTS

Week 1 15 minutes -- 3 days per week
Week 2 15 minutes -- 3 days per week
Week 3 20 minutes -- 3 days per week
Week 4 25 minutes -- 3 days per week
Week 5 25 minutes -- 3 days per week
with 1 lb hand weights
Week 6 25 minutes -- 4 days per week
Week 7 30 minutes -- 4 days per week
with 2 lb hand weights
Week 8 35 minutes -- 4 days per week
Week 9 35 minutes -- 4 days per week
Week 10 40 minutes -- 4 days per week
Week 11 40 minutes -- 4 days per week
Week 12 45 minutes -- 4 days per week

Table 5–B

you feel you're proceeding at a window-shopping pace, speed it up a bit. Many of the benefits of aerobic exercise are achieved at a moderate pace. You may find indoor "mall walking" to be particularly pleasurable during extreme weather conditions. Remember, "no pain - no gain" is a myth.

CHAPTER 6

PERSONALITY, LIFESTYLE, AND YOUR HEALTH

This chapter will explore what makes up our personality and the overlapping area, lifestyle — all the things we do. Certain personalities and lifestyles seem to go along with healthy lives; others go with unhealthy lives. If you are in the latter category and want to get out, is there anything you can do about it?

To answer that question, this chapter will define personality and lifestyle, and in particular, examine the behavior that makes up the "Type A personality."

PERSONALITY

Your way of perceiving and responding to the world generally remains relatively unchanged over the years. At your 10th or 25th high school or college reunion, you might not recognize your friends right away if their weight, hair, or faces have been changed with time. But when they start talking, you realize they are the same as always — their personalities have not changed. Personality is a person's consistent and enduring pattern of perceiving, thinking, feeling, and acting.

Personality develops early. Traits that can be observed in the first few weeks of a child's life become permanent parts of their personality. A selfish, whining, complaining child will become a selfish, whining, complaining adult. And not only is the pattern set, often so is a specific, life-long commitment. More than one adult has made such a statement as. "I marvel at the fact that a 17-year-old kid decided that I would become a surgeon."

106

LIFESTYLE

Lifestyle is everything we do. Lifestyle means more than where the "rich and famous" vacation and with whom they cavort. We may not have the power to carry out such a fantasy, but when it comes to health, you control all of the important aspects of your own lifestyle. You choose whether to smoke, bake in the sun, eat steak and fries, laze around, and just about everything else that affects your health.

You can limit these and other unhealthy behaviors, but most people don't. Why?

PERSONALITY AND LIFESTYLE

Personality and lifestyle not only overlap, many times they seem to be the same. Drinking excessive amounts of alcohol and eating a rich fatty diet describes a type of lifestyle, made up of behaviors determined by your personality. If we say that a person has a "devil-may-care" personality, we are also describing their behavior and lifestyle.

Now let's see just how much lifestyle contributes to, or controls the leading causes of death.

10 LEADING CAUSES
OF DEATH

Estimated Percent
Contribution
to Cause of Death

Table 6-A	LIFESTYLE	ENVIRONMENT	HEALTH CARE SERVICES	BIOLOGICAL
DISEASE				
1. Heart diseases	54%	9%	12%	25%
2. Cancers	37%	24%	10%	29%
3. Stroke	50%	22%	7%	21%
4. Motor vehicle accidents	69%	18%	12%	1%
5. Other accidents	51%	31%	14%	4%
6. Influenza/Pneumonia	23%	20%	18%	39%
7. Diabetes	34%	0%	6%	60%
8. Suicide	60%	35%	3%	2%
9. Cirrhosis	70%	9%	3%	18%
10. Homicide	63%	35%	0%	2%
All 10 averaged	51%	19%	10%	20%

Source: Center for Disease Control

The second column of Table 6-A, "Lifestyle," shows that in seven of the ten leading causes of death, over 50 percent of the risk factors are lifestyle-related. The three areas emphasized by this book — nutrition, exercise, and stress reduction — are precisely the ones where healthful choices can make a life-and-death difference.

In fact, in July of 1992, the American Heart Association upgraded physical inactivity from its list of "contributing factor" for cardiovascular disease to the stronger category of "risk factor." This places a sedentary lifestyle on par with high blood pressure, smoking, and high blood cholesterol.

Combined with other behaviors — alcohol consumption, smoking, and gaining excessive weight (fat) — this means that you can control most of the risk factors for those diseases that could cause you suffering and end your life prematurely. Can you change your lifestyle? Yes you can.

THE TYPE A PERSONALITY

Type A's are all around us; in fact they are just the type of person you want to have working for you. They move at full throttle, feeling they must do everything themselves. They take on more and more responsibility and get the job done NOW. They need to *have more, collect more, be more*; they feel a strong need for money and the things money will buy, as well as a strong need for praise and encouragement. They speak with energetic gestures, and a strong belief in what they are saying, and sometimes their ideas come out almost too fast for the words to be formed.

The Type A adult began exhibiting these behaviors somewhere around age 6 to 10. The Type A child even reacts physiologically like their adult counterparts; their heart rate and blood pressure elevate in response to challenges. By adulthood, these Type A patterns of internal and external responses have become automatic and consistent.

These Type A qualities are valued by employers, and Type A individuals are generally productive and well-adjusted. But one key attribute makes being a Type A a major health risk: *hostility* — the quick, high flying, free-floating anger which is closely related to coronary heart disease.

We are all impatient at times, but the Type A is impatient all the time; to the Type A, any perceived failure is devastating. They must be effective, must do better and more than anybody else; they must go around, or through, every obstacle. When healthy

110

aggression turns into free-floating hostility, effectiveness suffers and the Type A moves closer to the coronary care suite.

As we might expect, Type A behavior is often accompanied by smoking and hypertension. But the hostile Type A's, even if they lack these two risk factors have a higher rate of coronary heart disease.

IS THE TYPE A's FATE SEALED? NOT NECESSARILY

Personality traits endure because most of us make no significant effort to change them. Those who do *wish* to change don't usually do much more than that — wish. It has been demonstrated that behavior interventions can decrease Type A behavior and the rate of recurrent heart attacks in heart patients.

How can you change Type A behavior? It takes a concerted, committed effort and cannot be done in a week. Too bad — the Type A would like to accomplish this in the next hour. But as in dieting, short-term efforts don't work. Type A's need a fundamental change in the way they think, feel, and act.

In a five-year study (Friedman, et al, 1986) over 1000 heart-attack patients discussed with counselors their beliefs and values relating to their Type A behavior, and were assigned drills (such as eating more slowly, and smiling more — practices typically not followed by Type A's), given relaxation training, and taught to restructure their demands at work and at home. They also received cardiology counseling.

These patients had fewer future heart attacks than other Type A patients who received only cardiology counseling, or no treatment.

This improvement may have resulted from a reduction of the stress level, as well as the behavioral interventions, and may have been helped by the increased social support during the time of the experiment.

It should be no surprise that *smiling* reduces stress — for the smiler and smilee. When you are genuinely smiling, relating, or saying a kind word to someone, you cannot be experiencing a stress reaction. The two behaviors are incompatible. Also, think of the stress which is reduced if we simply *eat more slowly*, remain at the table for awhile and relax. And learn to *laugh* — at yourself, at life. It could save your life. And keep doing it.

Drilling and practicing can be essential. A good backhand stroke will disappear if you don't practice it. It is the same when replacing Type A behaviors with more beneficial, healthful behaviors. It is an ongoing, everyday process. Drop the old, use the new — for your heart's sake.

TAKE CONTROL

We have known for many years of the psychosomatic disorders where the mind influences the body in a negative way. The other side of the coin is that the mind can be used in positive ways to strengthen the body or to cure illnesses. And why not? The brain has approximately 100 billion nerve cells, many times the capacity of the most sophisticated computer.

We have huge stores of information in our brains. Even information we have temporarily forgotten is stored in there somewhere. It is in fact possible that somewhere in our brains is everything we ever learned, saw, felt, smelled, tasted, or heard.

In the following sections we are going to show how powerful the brain is, and how this power is being used to regain health for "hopeless" cases.

THE POWER OF THE BRAIN

A mental disorder that demonstrates not only the immense capacity and complexity of the human brain but also the startling amount of control it has over the body is called *multiple personality disorder* (MPD). In MPD (as shown in *The Three Faces of Eve* and *Sybil*) one person becomes someone else, like a Dr. Jekyll and Mr. Hyde, or becomes three, or dozens of different people, one at a time.

While some alleged cases of MPD have been shown to be fake — based on fantasy or fraud — most professionals agree that MPD is genuine. Approximately 6000 cases have now been diagnosed in the United States alone.

Besides different personalities, different physiologies appear. Susan may develop a rash when she drinks citrus juices. If a second, non-allergic, personality comes out while Susan has the rash, the itching may quickly go away and the rash may fade. One personality may be left- and another, right-handed; one nearsighted and one farsighted; some artistic, others not. Heart rate, respiration, and brainwave patterns may be different. A patient undergoing withdrawal from heroin, may show no withdrawal symptoms when changing to a different personality.

In some cases, a therapist can make a particular personality "come out." But usually, the personalities come out "involuntarily" in response to stress. MPD seems to originate in abuse during childhood. The child "escapes" by forming other personalities to take the punishment. Future personalities may be formed in response to later traumas. This "dissociation" is a form of self-hypnosis. The child learns to create, through hypnosis, a new more adaptive personality. MPD's are not only proficient at self-hypnosis, they are excellent hypnotic subjects — able to call forth any of the personalities when the therapist asks for "it." They are able to remember each mental state and keep them separate — to evoke them when needed.

This affinity for *hypnosis* is highly significant, when combined with their extraordinary control over the immune system. Roughly 25% of MPD's have personalities with differing allergic symptoms; about half have personalities that respond differently to the same medication; and, some personalities feel no pain at all.

If nothing else, this proves scientifically that the mind can both heal and destroy the body. Can the rest of us gain this healing ability?

Yes, many have, already. The same principles that allow the MPD's brains to organize and control are used by all of us every day. But we don't have the strength or motivation they have — the life-or-death situation that forces the young child to create new compartments and personalities. We can, however, learn to do some amazing things, as shown by the work of Dr. O. Carl Simonton, a radiation oncologist, and his ex-wife, Stephanie Matthews-Simonton, a psychotherapist.

BELIEFS, EXPECTATIONS, AND HEALTH

For many years the Simontons, working as a team, successfully used a traditional medical approach combined with psychological treatment. Their patients experienced double the national survival rate, and many were completely cured. Most of their patients had been identified as "medically incurable."

Carl Simonton learned as a young physician that his most successful cancer patients felt they did so well because they "had some reason to live." They felt they couldn't die because they were needed: "I can't die before my son graduates from college," or "not until I have solved this problem with my daughter." These cancer patients believed that they had some control over their disease — and therefore, they did.

Patients who believe they have no control, that only medical treatment can save them, whose doctors say that they have only a few months to live, usually die within the predicted time. It is the ones who decide to use all their internal resources for healing, who participate in the treatment and recovery process, who live.

What makes this possible? It is the will to live. It is not enough to say that you want to live — you have to mean it. Those patients who want someone or something to cure them, who are not working toward living, but are *cooperating in dying*, die.

The Simontons' treatment (in addition to traditional medical techniques) included teaching patients to relax, and teaching them to use *visualization* techniques. They were to visualize their cancer, whatever it looked like to them. Then they would visualize their radiation therapy as shooting millions of small bullets through the cancer cells and killing them. Then they created a mental image of the body's white blood cells swooping in and carrying off the dead cancer cells and flushing them out of the body through the liver and kidneys.

Not all of their patients completely eliminated their cancers and lived long and happy lives, yet some patients with "incurable" cancers did get rid of them. Others showed consistent progress such as the continued shrinking of a tumor, or a halt in the growth of the disease. However, some showed new tumor growth, and some died. But the overall success rate is impressive — especially considering that all these patients were regarded as medically incurable.

What the Simontons demonstrated is that patients can add to their years and to the quality of their lives by things they, the patients, do. The point is that the patients were using their minds to control processes in their bodies. These were not special patients who were selected because they were good at learning to visualize or to control their bodies. They were simply patients who wanted to live and who were willing to participate in their own treatment.

In the coming years you will be hearing about what is called the new science of *mental medicine*. This field should prosper because it allies ancient wisdom with recent research findings resulting from combining treatments for mind and body. It is one of many ways of describing the *mind-body connection*. Simply knowing the connection between mind and body states provides a starting point. Two examples of this symbiosis: among women with breast cancer that has spread to other parts of their bodies, those who participate in support groups survive twice as long; and a divorce has nearly the same impact on heart disease as does cigarette smoking!

Support groups offer positive emotional experience; divorce offers negative emotional experience, no matter how much you might want the divorce. The mind's state of health, its strength, its willingness and ability to fight can often be more important than the drugs or other treatments to the body. As the new strategies combining treatments for mind and body work successfully, the *mental* medicine approach to health care will undoubtedly grow.

CHAPTER 7

OBESITY AND PERSONALITY

Shelly Winters once quipped, "Where do you go to get anorexia?" But anorexia is no laughing matter. Too many people risk their health by trying to attain the unrealistic image of perfection created by society. Even anorexics who threaten their own lives by starving themselves, typically see themselves as fat.

Women are most affected by this — over half of all women are dissatisfied with their weight. In one survey (Winstead, et al, 1986), women in all weight-ranges were found to over-estimate their own weight status. Almost half of all underweight women thought they were "normal" or "overweight." And almost half of all women in the "normal" range thought they were overweight.

The problem of obesity, however, is not too much weight according to some charts, but too much fat. Football players are "overweight" by the charts but many have a very low percentage of body fat — they are overweight but not obese.

Clearly, heredity is one factor in obesity. When two people of the same age and sex, eating precisely the same diet maintain significantly different weights, we know that heredity is a factor — but it is just one factor. Rare disorders can cause extreme weight gain or loss, as in *myxedema* or in *hypothalamic tumors*.

MYXEDEMA, a thyroid condition leads to accumulation of fluids in the tissues, sluggishness, mental slowness, and weight gain. You can't fix this by yourself, but the condition can be treated by a physician, by using thyroid hormones.

A TUMOR of the ventromedial hypothalamus in the brain can cause a doubling or tripling of weight, in some rare cases. Destruction of one part of the hypothalamus causes excessive eating; destruction of another part causes undereating and weight loss.

These procedures have been used in animal research for years, and it is now technically possible to do the same for humans. But with the enormous risk involved and the possible legal complications, it will be awhile before the advent of the one-stop hypothalamus adjustment center in the shopping mall!

But, as mentioned, these are rare conditions, and most causes of obesity are largely within your control. Besides the survival need for food, we eat for many reasons; many of us eat two to four times as much as required for survival. We get used to that amount, and in effect, "overeat" just to feel right.

We also eat to be sociable. We load up on hamburgers, pizzas, all kinds of "junk food" as a part of our social lives. This means we eat the wrong, fat-filled foods, at the wrong time of the day — *no food should be eaten within four hours of going to bed.* Undigested food keeps the body working when it should be resting, and virtually no calories are burned off while we sleep. We then start the next day feeling groggy — and not especially hungry, so we skip the most important meal of the day, breakfast, and instead have some more health-wreckers — a couple of donuts and coffee at about 10 a.m.

We also eat when we are bored, depressed, happy, or sad — if you eat for emotional reasons there is always a "good reason" to eat.

But if we let our body do the talking, it will tell us when we are hungry and when we are not. Sensors in the liver detect sugar in the blood, but it takes about 20 minutes for the carbohydrates we eat to be converted to sugars in the bloodstream so that our sensors tell us we've had enough. By the time 20 minutes have passed, the obese have already eaten too much. Rapid eaters don't get the message soon enough — the simple change of EATING MORE SLOWLY will give the body a chance to tell you when it has had enough.

In general, the obese eat fewer meals per day, but eat more per meal, and they shovel it in faster than the non-obese. The amount on the fork is larger, the number of trips to the mouth is greater, and the time food stays in the mouth is less. Strangely, one doesn't leave good tasting foods in the mouth very long — the better it tastes, the faster it's swallowed.

Why hurry to get food to the stomach when the taste buds are all in the mouth? The answer is both psychological and physiological.

Psychologically, eating is enjoyable; it diverts our attention, and comforts us. Physiologically, any sweet or starchy foods increases the level of *serotonin*, a natural, necessary body chemical which has a calming effect. So, if we eat as a way of dealing with depression, we reward ourselves both psychologically and physiologically for feeling depressed, and so we gradually train ourselves to eat whenever we are depressed, tense, or angry.

There are other differences between the obese and the non-obese. Stomach contractions accompany hunger in the average person. But the obese are not as sensitive to these contractions — they are more sensitive to external cues, such as the sight or smell of foods. They eat available foods even if they have just eaten. If the food tastes good, they eat more. Their eating is less controlled by physical hunger, and more controlled by external stimuli — smell, taste, emotional situations.

People on diets, regardless of their weight, tend to behave like the obese. They respond more to external cues — probably because of the feeling, almost a panic, of being hungry. The food is there, so it is eaten, regardless of its nutritional value, or lack of it. Crackers, donuts, candy bars, whatever — down they go, slowed only by a fleeting sense of guilt.

Interestingly, the obese are less willing to work for food. In one experiment, non-obese subjects accepted almonds about half the time, whether they were shelled or unshelled. Obese subjects accepted shelled almonds almost all the time, but seldom the unshelled ones.

One final, obvious difference is that the obese are generally less active. It is a chicken-and-egg question: Does the extra weight cause lethargy or does inactivity cause the weight gain? The answer is, probably both.

Isn't it amazing that no animals in their natural habitats are fat? Animals are subject to genetic influence; they have diseases and disorders. But they don't get fat — unless we feed them. Hibernating animals add fat to carry them through the winter, but do not have excess fat at other times — they are too busy chasing food, or being chased. Humans in their natural environment don't get fat either. We have come a long way from our hunting-gathering days. We now live in an unnatural environment where unlimited food is available, and is constantly being offered to us. Where can you go where there is no food — shopping center, mall, movie, conference, meeting, gas station, a friend's house?

In the good-old-caveman days you might have had to walk or run for miles before you found a plant or animal for a snack or a meal. As great as that was for weight control, maybe we can find an easier way to arrive at and maintain a healthy weight.

BEHAVIORAL TREATMENT AND EATING

As mentioned above, the obese are very sensitive to outside stimuli or cues to eating. Anyone on a severely restricted diet becomes more sensitive to such stimuli. Therefore, behavioral treatment aims at controlling the stimuli, and thus the behavior. Stimuli that encourage overeating are gradually restricted, even eliminated.

For example, eating may be restricted to specific times or places. No eating is permitted while enjoying TV, movies, or other pleasures that tend to "double-up" with eating. Grocery shopping may be done only after eating, never when hungry.

Make notes of the stimuli that make you want to eat inappropriately. Do you pass a cookie shop on your way to the laundry? If so, take a different route. Do you snack on twinkies, cashews, pastries, chips? Don't bring them into the house. If you can't be trusted in the same room with a *Hershey* bar, don't bring it home. Instead, fill up the house with healthy snacks — keep a well-stocked fruit bowl.

In numerous studies, behavioral treatment of obesity has been found to be effective. One type of successful behavioral treatment (Mahoney, Moura, and Wade, 1973) provides rewards beyond weight reduction. The study involved five different groups:

1. A control group, which was given information about the study, but no treatment.

2. A self-monitoring group, which was asked to keep track of its weight each day.

3. A self-reward group, where the members were instructed to put aside a certain amount of money at each increment of weight loss. The money was to be used to buy things the individuals wanted.

4. A self-punishment group, in which individuals were fined if sufficient weight was not lost.

5. A combined self-reward/self-punishment group, using the procedures of both groups 3 and 4.

In the self-control groups (3, 4, and 5), the members were free to self-reward or self-punish as they saw fit, within the guidelines above. And it worked. Those in the self-reward groups (3 and 5) lost the most weight. Self-punishment was not an effective strategy, nor was simple weight monitoring, or just receiving guideline information. *The best results came from using self-rewards.*

You can reward yourself tangibly — by buying or doing something that you had been denying yourself. But intangibles, such as savoring the fact that you have succeeded in demonstrating control, are also rewards. Where might this "success" and demonstrated control lead?

Other studies show that behavioral treatment is superior even to the "social pressure" used in many weight-control programs. This is good news — it shows that your own ability to control your weight is more powerful than you had thought.

The hardest part is making up your mind to do it. Your motivation may increase when you learn that behavioral treatment not only produces excellent results in taking pounds off — it also produces important changes in your eating behavior. Studies also show significant improvement in the amount of "emotional and uncontrolled eating," "eating in isolation," "eating as a reward," and "between-meal eating."

Behaviorists say that if you change the symptom — the eating behavior — you solve the eating problem. The reason for the behavior is not important in this method — only the behavior itself. Other psychologists usually want to know "why" somebody does something, to deal with the underlying reasons for the behavior. Either approach can work well, but the behavioral approach is more practical and gets results faster — for obesity and for a whole range of other problems.

OBESITY AND FAD DIETS: MEETING THE EMOTIONAL NEEDS OF THE DIETER

Most of us know about Oprah Winfrey's diet efforts through the *Optifast*® program. ("Fast" has both meanings in the title.) In spite of her unlimited resources, Ms. Winfrey started regaining her lost weight shortly after she completed her diet, shortly after she proudly showed us her new figure in those impressive tight-fitting jeans. We were happy for her, but it didn't last long.

Yet, in spite of logic and scientific evidence, too many will try yet another fad diet. Why?

The first problem with fad diets involves self-worth and our media-dominated culture. We are taught that we are not worthy of being loved, admired, hired, promoted, or just BEING, unless we are as thin and "fit" as a *Vogue* or GQ model. Those of us who do not achieve the societal ideal easily fall prey to the promises of fad diets.

Our society has not always been so obsessed with thinness. In the 1940's and 1950's a somewhat fuller, "curvy" figure was considered ideal for women. Then in the '60s, the Parisian model became the ideal — Twiggy's boyish body with no breasts or curves. Actually achieving this ideal brings about dangerous changes in both the female psyche and metabolism.

A second reason fad diets are appealing is that we are obsessed with immediate gratification. We live in a fast-paced world where everyone wants everything NOW. Sound dietary programs cannot promise immediate drastic changes — so people turn to quick-fix fad diets.

Third, many people really don't want to change their eating habits on a long-term, way-of-life basis. A permanent behavior-modification approach to nutrition holds less appeal for most people than the rapid weight-loss promises of fad diets.

People too often diet for a particular short-term reason — to fit into a smaller dress for a wedding, to look great at the first summer beach party, to impress someone, or to convince your boss you're really ready for that big promotion — for any reason other than for a lifetime of wellness.

Finally, we like to talk about our "amazing progress" in a diet, to prove our self-worth by being better and faster than our peers. Who wants to race into the office and announce that they lost only one pound this week and only five pounds during the last month?

A friend of ours recently told us that her office had started a weight-loss competition. Everyone contributed money to a pool, and the biggest "loser" each week collected the money. We were horrified. This is exactly the type of program which leads to the yo-yo effect — and on a grand scale, with everyone in the office yo-yoing up and down. We hated to think of the emotional swings, the peer pressure, the subtle snobs and sniggers — the entire unhealthy, unhappy atmosphere being created.

As expected, there was short-term success, and long-term failure for the group as a whole. The only people who succeeded (happily, this included our friend) were those who had already committed to a long-term health and fitness program before the office competition began. For those few, the office pool was just an extra bit of fun.

If you are overweight, Mother Nature has a contract out on you. She is cruel in the short-term, but kind in the long-term. She wants to eliminate the problem now so that the genes are not passed on to future generations. The overweight develop diabetes, high blood pressure, and cancer more often than people of normal weight . Why pass these genes on? The overweight are less fertile, and therefore have fewer children. They can't jump out of the path of danger so easily, or even lift their own weight to save themselves. They die younger.

It should now be obvious that fad diets fit the lifestyles and emotional needs of too many people around the globe — for reasons that make them inevitably unsuccessful. Unfortunately, there is no magic. Long-term, healthy weight loss comes only through:

CONSISTENT
COMMITMENT
to
CHANGE

CHAPTER 8

EMOTIONS, PERCEPTIONS, AND HEALTH

We all know we have stress. And we all believe we have more than our fair share. When we say that we have a lot of stress, we speak as if we owned it, or as if it were a disease like measles or herpes. But stress is not a thing in the sense of a germ or a bug. In fact, some researchers say that stress doesn't exist — you can't point to it or show me where it is, so there is no such thing as stress. But stress is like beauty — in the eye of the beholder, or more accurately, in the *mind* of the beholder. Some people have a lot of stress and others have very little.

Stress is our physical response to a threat, or perceived threat. A stress response has three parts. The first is an *alarm reaction*, where our body mobilizes to meet the threat. The second stage is *resistance*, where we cope with or resist the stressor. The third phase, *exhaustion*, occurs if we are unable to resist successfully or eliminate the stressor. If stress is prolonged or repeated, we may suffer exhaustion and serious physiological damage.

This response to stress is a very primitive one. For the caveman, it was necessary for survival. The alarm state of, say, facing a saber-toothed tiger, gets him ready for "fight or flight." The sympathetic nervous system stimulates those functions needed for the emergency, and inhibits those that aren't. Heart rate and blood pressure are increased, and blood flow increases to the muscles but decreases to the skin. The bronchi in the lungs dilate to admit more air, while the blood vessels to the stomach and intestines constrict. The adrenal cortex releases corticosteroids, which give us access to protein, fat, and sugar for energy and decrease inflammation. All of the organs in the body are affected within a matter of seconds, and we are ready for anything.

But what usually happens in the modern world is that we are not required to face tigers, or any other real and immediate threat to our life or well-being. We are, nevertheless, subjected to stressors virtually every day, which call forth all of these reactions.

Being cut off in traffic, having the boss yell at you, hearing that someone has criticized you or your work, not getting the raise that you expected — any one of these can call forth the full alarm response which sets your sympathetic nervous system and your endocrine system into action. You are physically ready to fight or to run, but have no opportunity to do either. You simply sit in the traffic jam or look at the paycheck in disbelief, but seldom engage in the massive activity that your body is prepared to deliver.

The result is physical damage. Without a work-out, the muscles remain engorged with blood much longer, the blood pressure remains high, and clots may form in the blood vessels; blood flow to parts of the heart, lungs, or brain may be decreased or blocked completely. Death may result under any of these conditions.

THE MIND-BODY EFFECT

First, in a stress reaction, the brain becomes aware of a situation. It responds by calling for the release of a substance, which in turn causes changes in bodily reaction. These reactions then have additional effects on the brain. Mind affects body and body affects mind.

As we think about something, we evaluate, interpret, and determine what it means to us. We decide if it is something that calls for the stress reaction or not. But the same events or objects do not mean the same thing to all people, or even to the same person under different circumstances.

Driving behind a bus in heavy traffic on a cold rainy day, inhaling its exhaust, and being unable to see around it — your opinion of that bus may be unprintable! But to a shivering, wet person waiting on the next corner, it may be the most welcome sight in the world. The bus gives stress to one, and great relief to another. But it isn't the bus; it's the meaning the bus is given by the individual.

As an exercise, we asked undergraduate students to list all the negative outcomes of failing a major examination. Then we asked them to list real or

138

imagined positive outcomes. One student failed a test for a job she desperately wanted; she was crushed, but because of the failure, decided to go to college and raise her sights higher. She now sees that "failure" as one of the best things that ever happened to her.

Another failed the final in a course he had been barely passing. When he took the course again, for some reason "everything clicked." The course, which he had previously thought was "the pits," was now interesting, challenging, even exhilarating, and he got a B.

These are two examples of benefits resulting from failure — because of a positive attitude and determination to benefit even from a negative experience.

Some of us experience failure and stress *in spite* of what we do, others *because* of what we do. The latter — what we do to ourselves — is the source of most of our stress.

As an exercise, write down some of the things which cause you stress. Look at these items. How many of them have you created yourself? For example, if you wrote "not enough time," what does that mean? Not enough time to do what? List the things you would do had you more time. Which ones *must* you do? Who says? Which ones do you really *want* to do? Really? What value do these tasks or activities have for you? What will you gain by doing them, or lose by not doing them? One year, ten years from now, will you feel that this was a valuable or even a reasonable way to spend your time?

We all have 24 hours every day — kings, presidents, you, me, and bag-ladies. To make the best use of our time, it is helpful to remember theologian Reinhold Niebuhr's *Serenity Prayer*, whose power and common sense remain undiminished:

> *"O God, give us grace to accept with serenity the things that cannot be changed, courage to change the things which should be changed, and the wisdom to distinguish the one from the other."*

Some people we know have stopped reading or watching the news because it is too upsetting to them. Too many things in the world seem to need changing, yet they feel powerless to change them. So they stopped exposing themselves to the stress they associate with the news. For them, this stress-reduction technique works.

Others have chosen a political or environmental cause, and are determined to do something about that one thing. Writing to congressmen and newspapers, joining a group of like-minded people, raising funds, speaking — whatever their inclination and ability allow giving purpose and a sense of control, reducing their stress while accomplishing a noble goal.

STRESS AND DISPLACED AGGRESSION

What happens if we can't deal constructively with all the potential energy of a stress reaction? Let's say that your boss criticizes you unfairly at work. For many reasons, you can't respond as you would like to, so you stew all day, and by the time you get home, your spouse greets you and your response is X-rated. Your spouse wonders, "What did I say?" The answer of course, is nothing. This is *displaced aggression* — aggression directed to the wrong person.

When we don't have an appropriate outlet for aggression, we use whatever we can find. When we can't find someone else — or are too fair-minded to look — we turn it inward.

141

It is probably for this reason Matsushita Electric Industrial Company of Osaka, Japan, set up a room designed to promote harmony by allowing employees to vent their feelings. In the room is a portrait of the big boss, along with punching bags and stuffed figures for the employees to hit with their fists or bamboo sticks. They take out their frustrations in the room, and then return to work. Reports are that they go back to their jobs much calmer and happier after a few minutes in the "human control room."

Similar arrangements have been suggested for sales personnel in the U.S.A. One department store chain planned to place small rag dolls behind the counters, so that after an especially frustrating encounter with a customer, the salesperson could take out the doll and work it over. However, management dropped the plan out of fear that customers would find out why the salespeople were enjoying themselves so much!

But the principle is sound. Once the stress reaction kicks in, the best way to work off that energy is with *physical activity*. Running, hitting a punching bag, kicking a soccer ball — anything to work out those muscles and take the pressure off will make us feel better, and quickly return our systems to normal.

What are your major stressors? What causes you to get wound up tight? Your boss? Slow moving traffic? Someone leaving the top off the toothpaste? It doesn't have to be something that would make the 6 o'clock news. It is usually the little things that become "the last straw." Write down on a separate sheet of paper the things that have made you want to strangle someone or put your fist or foot in the appropriate place. Continue this list and keep it in this book for reference. We'll talk later about how to deal with these and other stressors.

STRESS AND BLOOD PRESSURE

Major stressful events and seemingly insignificant everyday hassles, along with real or imagined fears, can all cause the same physiological response. Let's think about stress and blood pressure. Whenever the stress response occurs, blood pressure increases, and then goes back to normal after a time, as illustrated in Figure 8-1. If, after awhile, we are stressed again, the blood pressure once again elevates and in time returns to the baseline.

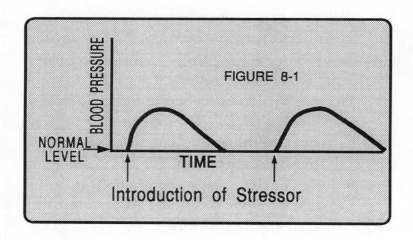

FIGURE 8-1

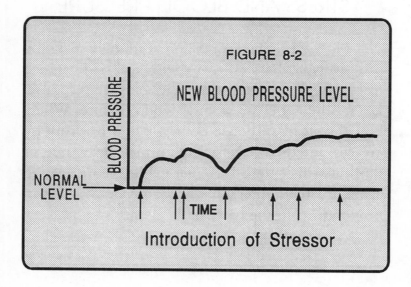

FIGURE 8-2

But if the stresses come closer together we may not fully recover from the first stress when the second occurs, so our blood pressure would not have returned to normal and would be pushed up yet higher, as in Figure 8-2. A third stressful event would push it even higher. A series of stresses close in time keeps our blood pressure at a high level.

In time, the blood pressure assumes a permanent, higher level — a higher unhealthy baseline. It doesn't take a whole series of insults for this to happen — all we have to do is to keep *thinking* about a single one, and we stress ourselves over and over again.

STRESS, ILLNESS, AND DEATH

Repeated stress causes headaches, stomachaches, overeating or overdrinking, smoking, ulcers and other psychosomatic problems, and virtually any other disease or disorder you might want to mention. Most have been shown to be caused or aggravated by stress.

If we compare ten major causes of death at the beginning of this century (Table 8-A) with known causes today, we can see what stress and lifestyle have to do with disease. The primary cause of the diseases italicized in the *Today* chart is lifestyle. Lifestyle refers

PRIMARY CAUSES OF DEATH

Table 8-A

1900

DISEASES	PERCENTAGE
Influenza and pneumonia	11.9%
Tuberculosis	11.4%
Gastroenteritis	8.4%
Heart disease	8.1%
Stroke	6.3%
Nephritis	4.8%
Accidents	4.3%
Cancer	3.8%
Diseases of infancy	3.7%
Diphtheria	2.4%
All others	34.9%

TODAY

DISEASES	PERCENTAGE
Heart disease	29.8%
Cancer	25.4%
Stroke	5.3%
Accidents, including motor vehicles	12.7%
Lung disease, emphysema, asthma, and bronchitis	3.7%
Pneumonia and influenza	2.6%
Diabetes mellitus	2.2%
Suicide	2.2%
Chronic liver disease & cirrhosis	1.7%
Human immunodeficiency, virus infection (HIV)	1.7%
All other causes of death	12.7%

to the choices we make and the things we do. Do you smoke, drink, eat plenty of animal fat, and drive without seatbelts? These are your choices. It is you who decides to stay up all night, go without breakfast, forget exercise, and get sunburned. The consequences are shown in the *Today* chart. These activities all put stress on your system; physiological and/or emotional stress, which figures prominently in almost all of today's major causes of death.

Note that all of the listed causes of death are italicized except for one category — pneumonia and influenza. Look at each cause of death and think about what you might be doing to get yourself listed in that statistic. No, you can't control all of the factors, but you will discover that your choices, your behavior, have much to do with your state of health.

Also note that almost three-quarters of deaths are attributable to the first four categories — heart disease, cancer, stroke, and accidents. Now let's see whether we can delay death to a reasonable time by avoiding the conditions and illnesses that lead us to it prematurely.

In 1967, Holmes and Rahe looked at events in people's lives to see whether there was any relationship between the number of changes in one's life and subsequent illness. They listed 43 events including: death of spouse, divorce, marriage, fired at work, death of close friend, outstanding personal achievement, change in residence, and vacation. Respondents were to check all events that had occurred in their lives in a given time period. Later versions of the scale weighted the items because it was obvious that death of a spouse, for example, was far more stressful than a change in residence. Still, any change or adjustment adds something to the total load of stress.

Respondents with high scores became ill more frequently than those with low scores. Other researchers have verified the connection between *the amount of change required in one's life* (one definition of stress) and subsequent illness such as infectious disease, metabolic disturbances, or heart disease.

Following the loss of a job, some people experience an increase in blood pressure, ulcers, and swollen joints. Others show signs of diabetes and atherosclerosis soon after losing their jobs. Yet many show mild or no effects.

KOBASA AND STRESS

This leads to some very interesting work by Suzanne Kobasa, who discovered that people's ability to cope with stress depends on their *"level of hardiness."*

Kobasa was interested in finding out the importance of personality as a factor in stress-linked disorders. Are there characteristics of our personality that will make a stressful situation even worse? And are there characteristics or traits that will help minimize stress? Her study indicated that many people exposed to extraordinary stresses do not become ill.

Kobasa's work identified several factors associated with good health in the face of extreme stress. They can be stated in three words: *Control, Commitment,* and *Challenge.*

Those with a greater sense of *control* over their lives remain healthier in the face of stressful events. They feel that they can make decisions, choose what to do — and when stressful situations occur, react with appropriate responses, realizing that stress is a part of life that must be addressed. Those with no sense of control instead adopt a hopeless, helpless attitude. They feel powerless and unmotivated, out of control, unable to cope, and these are the ones who become stressed to the point of mind or body illness.

Commitment means having a stake in what you do, and a stake in being involved with others. This provides meaning and motivation for the struggle when times get tough. Being committed to one's family, work, church, or community is important in remaining healthy in the face of stress. And so is commitment to yourself — knowing what you want, your values and goals, and carrying them out, one by one.

The third characteristic, *challenge*, refers to how you view change. Those who accept change and look forward to it as a challenge and an exciting part of life are much more likely to remain healthy than those who see change as a threat. To stay healthy, welcome change as the giver of new experiences, new challenges, new growth, as the key to new doors, new vistas, new opportunities.

Control, commitment, and challenge make up what Kobasa calls "*hardiness,*" the trait which enables people to deal with stress effectively.

Those who become ill, by comparison, have reduced self-esteem, a sense of isolation or few social relationships, and a low level of gratification from interpersonal interaction. They exhibit the "*giving up-given up"* syndrome. Lacking control, commitment, and challenge, they have no defenses against stress.

This research shows what behaviors and attitudes are associated with healthy versus unhealthy lives. But can we translate these findings into practical use? How do we fight stress, or decrease the amount of stress we experience, avoid stressful situations, or deal with the inevitable stress we experience?

The next chapter will deal with these issues and give suggestions based on extensive research on lifestyle as well as stress itself.

CHAPTER 9

STRESS BUSTERS

The most frequently prescribed drugs of the 1980's and 1990's were an ulcer medication, a hypertension drug, and a tranquilizer. All of these treat symptoms of stress caused by worry, anxiety, nervousness, tension, or pressure. Doctors, being sympathetic, prescribe drugs to eliminate or decrease these symptoms, but drugs are never the best way to treat stress. They do nothing for the underlying cause of the symptoms, so even if the drugs are not literally habit-forming, their continued use, often in ever-increasing doses, is necessary to prevent the symptoms.

It is surprising how many patients report they are not taking any drugs, yet on further questioning, admit that they do take *Valium*, but don't consider it a drug. They could stop if they wanted to, but feel better when they are taking it. Of course the problem is that they keep taking it because they don't like the withdrawal symptoms when they stop. Other anti-anxiety medications such as *Librium*, *Ativan*, and *Xanax*, also have long-term side effects and the potential for withdrawal problems.

Some drugs, such as *insulin* for diabetics, are prescribed for a lifetime, because there is no existing cure, so the alternative is more dangerous than accepting *insulin's* potential dangers and side effects. But most drugs are intended to be used for only a *short time*, to prevent or cure an illness, or to relieve symptoms.

Taking drugs to relieve symptoms can be useful in the short-term, until the body heals itself, or until the condition causing the symptoms is no longer present (allergy season passes, the bruised bone heals, the visiting relatives go home). It is the long-term unnecessary use of drugs that should be discouraged.

A far better way to treat the symptoms of stress is to treat the underlying cause of the symptoms — the stress itself.

This chapter considers a number of relaxation techniques that can provide the stress reduction you might otherwise seek through drugs. Learning relaxation techniques is like getting a vaccination — it prepares you for stress, and shields you from its negative effects. You will also learn how to relax in the middle of a stressful situation.

For certain stresses, you may want to consider making some lifestyle changes to eliminate the things in your life that create the stress — actually eliminating the root causes. But since you can never eliminate all sources of stress in a normal life, these seven stress-buster exercises treat the symptom effectively and healthfully, and they have no adverse side effects.

1. LAUGHING STRESS AWAY

Norman Cousins describes in his book *Anatomy of an Illness* how he got relief from excruciating and unremitting pain by cultivating a full-blown, out-loud belly laugh. He checked himself out of the hospital and into a hotel, where he watched films of his favorite laugh-provoking shows. He was able to sleep, when medications had failed to provide either pain relief or sleep. Laughter apparently decreases the production of *adrenaline*, one of the hormones released when we are under stress. Incidentally, coffee or alcohol, or smoking cigarettes *increases* adrenaline.

Develop your own ways of stimulating your humor. View situations in different ways. When faced with a problem, try to see the positive side, the benefit, the funny side. The more you practice, the easier it gets. In time, you will learn to control not only your problems and your reaction to them, but your internal state. Remember Aristotle's definition of the difference between tragedy and comedy: In tragedy, you take the short view, and are immersed in it; in comedy you take the large view, where you are able to see the humor in it.

2. BREATHING STRESS AWAY

Most people have never learned how to breathe. Ask someone to take a deep breath and the chest expands and rises; the shoulders lift; and the stomach goes in. This kind of deep breath not only doesn't relax you, but causes more tension in the back, neck, and shoulders, which can lead to headaches, vision problems, stiffness and tightness in the chest, shoulders and neck.

Then, how should we breathe? Try this: Lie down on your back, and place one hand on your chest, the other hand on your stomach; breathe normally. For most people, the chest hand rises during inhalation and falls during exhalation. The stomach hand will fall as you inhale, because as the chest expands the stomach pulls in. This is probably the way you have always done it, but it is *wrong*.

In *proper* breathing, the lungs expand by expanding the stomach. The diaphragm, a large muscle below the lungs, drops to allow the lungs to expand downward. The chest moves only slightly as you exhale. When you breathe properly, therefore, the stomach hand *rises as you inhale* and falls as you exhale. The chest hand either doesn't move at all, or moves slightly IN THE SAME DIRECTION as the stomach hand.

Look in a mirror and take a deep "relaxing" breath. If your shoulders rise or your stomach goes in, you are creating tension, not relaxation. Practice pushing your stomach out to allow lung expansion, and you will see that your shoulders and chest do not rise. This is correct breathing, but if you aren't used to breathing this way, it will feel awkward at first.

When you lie down to relax, put your hands on your chest and stomach to make sure your breathing is easy and natural. Train yourself so that the relaxed way of breathing becomes a normal part of your life. After you have learned, you may require only occasional checks when you're feeling tense to bring back this healthful rhythm.

3. SOAKING STRESS AWAY

A bath? No, a warm soak — no soap, no scrubbing. Just make the water body-temperature or slightly higher (98 - 100 degrees); put a towel or tub pillow behind your head, close your eyes, and relax. Think of floating on a pink cloud, lying in the sun on a deserted beach. Stay as long as you want, even a short soak sometimes works wonders.

4. WALKING STRESS AWAY

Moderate exercise tones the muscles and the nervous system. After only a 20-minute walk, your muscles and nerves will be at a more relaxed state for an hour or two. This is similar to the progressive relaxation techniques outlined later in this chapter — tensing muscles, then relaxing them. The restful effects of walking persist long after the walk has ended. If you haven't time for a walk, put on music for a few minutes, and move — your body will be resuscitated, and so will your mind.

5. KNOWING WHEN TO SAY NO

Social gatherings can be enjoyable and productive — or debilitating. Some people use them to ask for unfair favors, or to pass on responsibilities while both of you are impaired by alcohol.

The person who wants something, and passes the responsibility to you by saying "Call me," has put you in the position of calling them for something they want. Of course, if you will benefit from it, make the call. But why should you put out the effort which is clearly the responsibility of, and which will only benefit, the other person?

Every time you accept responsibility to "Call, won't you?" you are accepting a necklace — a rock on a rope — that you must wear until you do what you promised. After accepting a number of these requests — "Will you take care of that?" "Let me hear from you next week," — your neckwear starts getting pretty

159

heavy. Even when you go to bed, it's still there — a pain in the neck, which adds to your stress.

What can you do? Don't accept the rock! Sometimes you can see them coming. The conversation starts with the weather, the stock market, or your new clothes, and then, suddenly, "Oh by the way..." And here comes a horror story, or a rock, or both: "By the way, was it your department that hired that serial killer? We were wondering what you're going to announce to ease everyone's mind."

It is not just cocktail parties — offices are favorite rock-distribution sites. Your boss hands out rocks and you accept them; that's your job, if the boss gives the right rock to the right person. But sometimes it is the subordinate who hangs the rock on the boss.

Some years ago I received a promotion, and the psychiatrist who was director of the Health and Counseling Center called me and said, "Congratulations. I see you're my new boss." I was pleased; we were friends and generally saw things the same way; it would be a pleasure working with him.

Then he added, "Now here's what I want you to do for me." Wow, that didn't take long! I had naively assumed that I would be telling *him* what he could do for me, or for the organization. But after listening, I decided he was correct — these were important needs for that center. But I suggested that he formalize his requests in writing so I could consider his rocks along with everyone else's. Taking on a neck-load of rocks was part of my job — accepting them over the phone was not.

So know when it is your rock to accept. If it's not, just say no!

6. DEVELOPING A NON-STRESSFUL ATTITUDE

Whenever you miss a shot in tennis, do you say, "dummy," or "you jerk," because you should have made it? A better approach is to analyze why you missed it: "Should have bent my knees..." and then do it right away; bend your knees, and take the proper swing. Correcting the problem helps; destructive criticism does not. Even mild negative comments sink into your brain, and accumulate. Why do that to yourself?

Consciously and unconsciously, we have been collecting and carrying destructive messages all our lives. Parents, teachers, other children told us, "I hate you." "You'll never amount to anything." "You're no good ...ugly ...stupid... fat..." Whether these statements have any basis in fact does not matter. They were said, they were heard, they went into your head, they stayed there, and they influence your behavior today; they help make up your self-concept.

Give yourself positive messages, "I have confidence in myself... I am intelligent, resourceful, happy, optimistic. I can always see something positive in any situation. I can achieve what I want to achieve." Review your strengths, and write them down, along with what you would like your strengths to be. Complete the sentence, "I feel best about myself when I..." List a number of endings and then do those things. Start with modest goals and achieve them. Make the list grow.

7. BEING TRUTHFUL

Don't lie and don't do anything about which you will have to lie. This is not only sound moral advice, it will remove a major load of stress. If you never lie, you won't have to worry about keeping your stories straight, or about being caught in your lie.

The same holds for actions — if you are comfortable with your actions, you need have no discomfort discussing them.

When we act or speak in opposition to our beliefs or values, we suffer stress which will persist until our beliefs and behaviors coincide.

PRAYER

There is no right or wrong way to pray; no particular words must be used. To reduce stress, make your own prayer, use your own words, rather than reciting or reading someone else's. The prayer must have meaning for you. You do not have to consider yourself a religious person, or even attend church to use prayer effectively. And, like most other human endeavors, the more you use prayer, the easier, more enjoyable, and more effective it becomes.

MEDITATION

If someone tells you to relax, what do you do? Do you sit down with a cigarette, or a cup of coffee, or both? Do you get angry? Do you try to sit still and "do nothing?"

But how do you "do nothing?" It's like being told: "Concentrate on not thinking about an elephant."

Our minds are always working, and so are our bodies — always breathing, pumping blood, sending nerve transmissions, repairing injuries, cleaning out toxic substances, using our major and minor muscle groups to shift various parts of our body around.

So it is impossible to completely shut down either the mind or the body, but it is possible to engage in healthful, restful activity for each.

First, we want to learn to control our thoughts. Since we can't clear everything from the mind, let's decide on what will be there. We can make our minds effectively clear if we concentrate on just one thing. And if that thing has no particular emotional meaning to us, we are relaxed. One way to meditate is to keep repeating that thought or word, so that the mind is filled with just that one thing.

Meditators repeat a *mantra*, a word or phrase or sound, to exclude all other thoughts from the mind. This has worked effectively for centuries. And meditation is one of the easiest forms of relaxation to learn. We don't have to wrap ourselves in a turban and a king-sized diaper and sit cross-legged on a mountain — most of us are more relaxed, and better able to meditate, in a chair.

To meditate, find a place that is quiet, and where you won't be disturbed. Get comfortable. Wear loose clothes or loosen any belts, straps, shoes — anything that you can feel putting pressure on any part of your body.

Now, think of the word "relax." Take a few deep (stomach-moving) breaths and mentally say "relax," as you let each breath flow out. Whatever word you have chosen, "relax," or "peace," or "one," say it to yourself; see the word; fill your mind with that word. If your mind wanders, don't worry about it, just get back to thinking of your word.

It will take practice, but try to work up to meditating for 15 minutes, twice a day. Most people feel that the best times are at the very beginning and at the very end of the day. Get up 15 minutes early so you won't feel rushed. The idea is to relax, not to cram one more thing into an already busy schedule. As in most things, the hardest part is in getting started. So start tonight.

PROGRESSIVE MUSCLE RELAXATION

This can be one of your greatest weapons against stress. Make a fist with your right hand, and tense all the muscles in your wrist and forearm. With your left

hand, squeeze various places along your right forearm and wrist, and feel the tightness of the muscles.

Now relax the right hand and let it fall open, and
let all the muscles go limp. Imagine all the tension
draining out through the fingertips. Notice the difference in this relaxed feeling and the earlier tensed
feeling. Note how soft and relaxed the muscles are
now. Throughout this exercise, breathe easily and
regularly.

You are now ready to apply tension-relaxation to
your entire body, in a slow, easy, enjoyable sequence.

Tense the muscles in your face. Frown, scowl,
make a "prune face" by forcing your lips forward like
a funnel. Do faces that tense all the muscles, and
don't forget the forehead and the muscles around the
eyes. It may take a few tries before you get most or all
of your facial muscles involved at once. Hold the face
tense for a few seconds, and then relax. Smooth out
the forehead, let the jaw drop, relax the eyes. Let the
tension drain out as you breathe deeply several times,
saying to yourself, "relax," each time you exhale.

Now, tense your neck, and after a few seconds,
relax. Take a moment to relax, breathing deeply and
regularly. Tension in the shoulders and neck can

bring on headaches at any time of day. If you realize that you are unconsciously tensing up, in the course of the day, you can immediately get rid of the tension.

Next, tense your upper arms and shoulders. Hold the tension for 5-6 seconds and then relax, letting the shoulders fall and all the tension run out. Continue with the lower arms and hands by making and releasing your fists; do both sides together. Go on to the stomach, thighs, lower legs, and feet. For the last, curve the toes down or up while stiffening the calf muscles. Push your feet against the floor if sitting, or against the wall or the arm of a couch if lying down. Feel the tension, then let it go, and relax.

Now, spend a few minutes searching your body for tight spots and relaxing them, one by one, all the while breathing as described earlier. Each time you exhale, say "relax," or "peace," or "I am relaxed."

Some people prefer to pause longer between muscle groups, taking 15-20 minutes for the whole body sequence. You may take less time, and later, you will learn to be selective, concentrating on your own particular tension spots. But the goal is not to do the exercises quickly; the goal is to relax, and that means not hurrying.

When you have completed tensing, then relaxing all parts of your body, rest comfortably, eyes closed, breathing easily, and saying "relax" with each exhalation.

SYSTEMATIC DESENSITIZATION OF FEARS

All of us fear something — snakes, spiders, the dark, crowds, your landlord, the government, blind dates. When a fear is out of proportion to the danger, then it is called a *phobia*. A person with a snake phobia might go into an uncontrollable panic at the sight or even the thought of a snake.

Fortunately, phobias can be successfully treated. One method is called *systematic desensitization*, where the patient is exposed to the feared object or situation in the least threatening way possible.

The subject is first taught a relaxation technique, such as progressive relaxation, and is then asked to visualize the feared object or situation — and at each step is asked to relax while thinking about the object of fear.

Sensors record muscle tension, skin conductance, heart rate, and other physiological measures to let the therapist and subject know when a sufficient level of relaxation has been reached, and then a *slightly* more threatening presentation is made.

When people rank their greatest fears, snakes come out near the top, along with speaking before a group. Here is the sequence that would be followed in desensitizing both of these fears.

FEAR OF SNAKES

1. Show the subject a still picture of a snake.

2. Show nature films or videos of snakes.

3. Show a snake in a glass case in an adjoining room.

4. Show a snake in a glass case in the same room.

5. Subject touches the glass case containing the snake.

6. Therapist handles the snake in presence of subject.

7. Subject touches the snake while therapist holds it.

8. Subject takes the snake from therapist, handles it, and returns it to the glass case.

9. Subject takes the snake from the case, handles it, and returns it to the case.

FEAR OF PUBLIC SPEAKING

1. The subject imagines speaking in front of a group.

2. Subject attends conferences, lectures, local meetings, and watches people speaking, and imagines himself or herself being the speaker.

3. Subject gives a speech into a tape recorder, while visualizing speaking to a group, then plays the speech back to a support group which is being trained to overcome the fear of speaking. It is important to pick a topic the subject knows well — the stress of speaking is enough, without the fear of being unprepared, and looking foolish.

4. Subject makes a brief presentation to the support group, using notes, or even reading the entire presentation.

5. Subject makes a brief statement at a public meeting, as a member of the audience.

6. Subject speaks to the support group without notes, developing, over time, eye contact, and appropriate gestures.

7. Subject speaks to other groups, moving on, over time, to larger and larger groups.

The sessions may take days or weeks, with the feared object or situation being presented in increasingly challenging ways, as the subject learns to relax at one level before moving on to the next. Some people breeze through the process, and others get stuck temporarily at one stage.

"Modeling," watching someone else handle a snake or speak publicly, demonstrates that the behavior is not harmful. The speaker did not faint, freeze up, or get attacked by the audience. The garden snake did not bite anyone.

Why does systematic desensitization work? The first reason has to do with the physical response — the object of fear makes the heart beat faster and digestion slow down. But when we relax, the heart slows down and digestion speeds up. We can't have it both ways at the same time, so learning to consciously call forth a relaxation response prevents the stress response from occurring.

The second way desensitization works is by forcing people to confront the object of fear and learn about it. Someone who fears snakes does not visit snake farms, or touch the pet snake of the kid next door. Someone with a fear of horses does not get on a horse, or even near one. They never have real-life proof that touching a snake or a horse is not life-threatening; their only experience with snakes or horses is their own fear — which is never contradicted by experience.

No matter what the fear or phobia, the same avoidance behavior reinforces the person's future behavior to continue avoiding that thing or that situation.

What stresses you? Have you tested it? Not just by getting close to it, but by grabbing it with both hands, by facing it fully and squarely? If the direct and immediate approach is too much, maybe your own creative version of systematic desensitization will work. If not, guidance from a professional will probably help.

BIOFEEDBACK

Checking your temperature or looking in the mirror to assess your weight are forms of biofeedback. So is any method you use to get objective information about what's going on in your body.

Sophisticated biofeedback equipment can make precise measurements of skin temperature, muscle tension, skin conductance, blood pressure, pulse, and other physiological functions.

A simple measure of overall relaxation is hand temperature. Warmer hands mean the person is more relaxed, has lower blood pressure, slower pulse, and more regular breathing. If you hold the bulb of a small thermometer between your thumb and forefinger, it will indicate your finger temperature. (Hand temperature should be checked in a comfortable room, around 70 degrees, otherwise room temperature will influence the reading.) If you relax, the blood vessels in your hands expand and carry more blood, raising the temperature. After a few days of practice, you can teach yourself to raise your skin temperature higher, in less time, with less effort.

Most thermometers measure temperature only in one or two degree increments, but electronic thermometers measure within one-tenth or one-hundredth of a degree. They provide immediate feedback on temperature changes, so you know that whatever you are doing at that moment is raising or lowering hand temperature — and therefore raising or lowering your tension level.

As a quick check to see if you're relaxed, touch your fingertips to the back of your neck. If your fingers feel cold, you are not relaxed. The back of the neck is consistently warm, whereas finger temperature can vary 10 degrees in a short period of time.

Great strides have been made in treating a variety of disorders with biofeedback. Dr. Steven Fahrion and others at the Menninger Foundation have been using biofeedback for years to teach hypertensives to monitor themselves during relaxation exercises. They have successfully decreased blood pressure to within normal limits, allowing patients to discontinue high blood pressure medication.

Biofeedback is also used to treat migraine head-aches, anxiety, and cardiac arrhythmias (irregular heart beats). It also works well with *Raynaud's disease*, in which cold weather or emotional stress causes con-tractions or spasms in the arteries in the hands or feet, sometimes actually turning them blue or white because of decreased circulation. Biofeedback, along with muscle relaxation or autogenic training, teaches one to relax and increase blood flow to the hands or feet.

Still other studies show biofeedback to be effec-tive in treating muscle-contractions, headaches, gas-trointestinal disorders, and incontinence. It is dramatically successful against urinary incontinence in older people, who are slow in receiving signals from their bodies, and may suffer from weakened muscles.

Biofeedback works only as part of the process of relaxation. The feedback merely helps the subject learn what to do to relax, and what not to do. As part of an effective relaxation strategy, biofeedback can work "miraculously" well.

AUTOGENIC TRAINING

Autogenic means "self-produced" and is a relaxation technique that emphasizes imagery and self-suggestion. It is a good technique that anyone can easily learn and enjoy. It resembles progressive muscle relaxation, except that thought alone is used to attain a calm and relaxed state, rather than physically tightening and loosening muscles. Autogenic training concentrates on your awareness of your body's heaviness, warmth, heartbeat, and breathing. Particular attention is given to the solar plexus and forehead.

Read this entire section before you decide exactly which sequence to follow. As in meditation, find a quiet place where you will not be disturbed, and make yourself comfortable. Your eyes will be closed (to eliminate visual stimuli) and you will be relaxed, but you will remain awake and aware of the words you are saying to yourself.

Start with the first category, *heaviness*, and when you have mastered that, move on to the next. You may need more or less time than suggested for each area, so move at your own pace. If you have difficulty with a particular part, go on to the next one and come back later.

At the end of a session, say to yourself, "When I open my eyes, I will be fully awake and feeling good." Then slowly open your eyes, take several deep breaths, and stretch your arms and legs.

The phrases can be used in many combinations. You may begin by using the exercises one at a time, in the order given, or you may combine HEAVI-NESS with WARMTH, etc., to go more quickly through the procedure. If you wish to extend the heaviness exercise beyond the legs and arms to all parts of the body in the first week or even the first day, that is okay too. Discover what works for you and how rapidly you want to proceed.

HEAVINESS

Repeat the statements below, slowly and silently. Start with your dominant arm — your right arm, if you are right-handed. Repeat each statement ("My right arm is heavy.") four to six times, and then move to the next statement:

My right arm is heavy.
My left arm is heavy.
Both arms are heavy.

Begin with one to five sessions a day, around two minutes each. Even on your busiest days, make sure you do something — even if only two or three 30-second sessions. As you gradually increase the length of each session to 30 or 40 minutes, you can cut the number to two sessions per day. When you have mastered all the exercises, you will be able to cut back again, and still achieve great benefits with two 10-15 minute sessions a day.

After the first week, move on to the next set of phrases:

My right arm is heavy.
My left arm is heavy.
Both arms are heavy.
My right leg is heavy.
My left leg is heavy.
Both legs are heavy.
My arms and legs are heavy.

If you find it hard to experience heaviness, imagine weights pressing down on your arms and legs. Feel the heaviness from your shoulder all along every part of your arm, down to your fingertips; from your hip joint all along your legs, down to your feet and toes.

WARMTH

In this section, concentrate on feeling warmth spreading throughout your body. You may have felt warmth during the heaviness exercises, and you may want to repeat the heaviness phrases before saying these:

My right arm is warm.
My left arm is warm.
Both arms are warm.
My right leg is warm.
My left leg is warm.
Both legs are warm.
My arms and legs are warm.

Imagine lying on a blanket in the sun, or having heating pads on your arms and legs. Picture yourself immersed in a warm tub of water, sipping your favorite hot drink. Visualize and feel your warm blood moving into your arms and legs, all the way down to your fingertips and to your toes.

HEARTBEAT

This exercise expands the warmth to the area of the heart:

My right arm is heavy.

My arms and legs are heavy and warm.
My heartbeat is calm and regular.

If you are not aware of your heartbeat and want to feel it, lie on your back with your head supported, and rest your hand over your heart.

BREATHING

Use relaxed stomach-breathing to enhance muscular relaxation and mental tranquility, as you repeat:
My right arm is heavy and warm.
My arms and legs are heavy and warm.
My heartbeat is calm and regular.
My breathing is calm and relaxed.

ABDOMINAL AREA (SOLAR PLEXUS)

My right arm is heavy and warm.
My arms and legs are heavy and warm.
My heartbeat is calm and regular.
My breathing is calm and relaxed.
My solar plexus is warm.

FOREHEAD

In this final exercise, we concentrate on *cooling* rather than warming. When blood flows to the arms and legs, and chest and solar plexus, it leaves the head. Therefore, it is best to practice this exercise lying down, and to do only a few repetitions the first time, to avoid dizziness.

My right arm is heavy and warm.
My arms and legs are heavy and warm.
My heartbeat is calm and regular.
My breathing is calm and relaxed.
My solar plexus is warm.
My forehead is cool.

If one week is devoted to each set of phrases, it will take seven weeks to incorporate all seven into your sessions. Since the phrases are cumulative, that is, you review the old and add the new, by the end of the seven weeks (more or less, depending on your pace) you will have completed the basic autogenic training sequence. From that point on, each relaxation session should include all of these last six phrases. With constant practice, you may find that within a few months, you can go through all the stages in five minutes or less, achieving the desired state of relaxation, warmth, heaviness, etc. Whenever you reach that point, stay in the state of autogenic meditation for 20 or 30 minutes. This is wonderfully healing to your body and mind.

LAST WORDS ON STRESS REDUCTION

That these techniques require time is actually a great advantage. When we practice them, we are substituting a period of relaxation for a period of stress. We are learning that we are worth some time. And we learn that the time was not really taken from us; instead, we become more productive, accomplishing more in less time. It has been known for decades that if people are given breaks from work, they accomplish much more in the course of a day than if they had worked all day without stopping.

These techniques provide a powerful arsenal of stress fighters. But you must master them to make them work for you, and that means *using* them. Knowing how to walk does you no good unless you get out and put your feet on the pavement. You must do it, not just know about it.

CHAPTER 10

REDUCING YOUR RISK OF
HEART DISEASE

The good news about heart attacks is that they are occurring at a lower rate today than in the 1950's and 1960's, partly because the causes of heart disease are better understood today than ever before, and many of us have learned to take steps to reduce our risk of heart disease. And the quality of treatment for cardiovascular disease has improved dramatically, with procedures such as balloon angioplasty and coronary artery bypass graft surgery.

The bad news is that heart disease is still the number-one killer in the world. But this doesn't have to be so — there are clear, understandable risk factors associated with heart disease, and some definite ways to improve your personal risk-factor profile.

THE MAJOR RISK FACTORS

Only a few risk factors for cardiovascular disease are beyond your control — family history, diabetes, male gender, and age. Most risk factors depend at least partly on your personal choices about lifestyle, and these factors also happen to be the most dangerous — cigarette smoking, hypertension, elevated cholesterol levels, lack of exercise, obesity, stress, second-hand smoke, and certain aspects of Type A behavior.

You could never eliminate all risk of heart disease. The objective is just to lower your overall risk, and there is a great deal you can do about that, especially if you understand that heart disease does not appear quickly; it is *several decades in the making*.

8 MYTHS ASSOCIATED WITH HEART DISEASE

As with most health issues, there are many myths about heart disease, and some of them are not only misleading but dangerous. Some are perpetrated by companies using misleading advertisements; others simply in the form of "common knowledge."

MYTH 1. INVULNERABILITY

You may believe that you won't have a heart attack if none of your close relatives has been an early victim. But the renowned, Framingham (Massachusetts) Study showed that, while a good family history is a positive factor, it cannot overcome the lifestyle dangers created by cigarette smoking, hypertension, high cholesterol levels, and obesity.

MYTH 2. HOPELESSNESS

Conversely, you may believe that if premature heart disease runs in your family you are destined to die at a young age of a heart attack, so it is useless to follow a heart-healthy lifestyle. Maybe you deliberately live an unhealthy lifestyle, in an effort to squeeze 100 years of living into a 40- or 50-year lifespan. But few families are 100% free of heart disease, and few have all members die of heart disease by age 40. The important lesson is that all of us can change the odds of developing heart disease at an early age, by attending to those risk factors which are under our control. If you have a family history of heart disease, examine the lifestyles of those early-death individuals. You will probably find that they contributed to it by the life they led.

MYTH 3. WONDER WOMAN

Some people believe that women don't have heart attacks. While it is true that premenopausal women have a distinct advantage over same-age men, cardiovascular disease is the number-one killer of postmenopausal women.

And young women can have heart attacks, too... although some young women and even their doctors don't seem to recognize this fact. Don't ignore symptoms simply because you are young and female. If you have any of the risk factors mentioned earlier, your risk increases with each one.

Women may surpass men for heart disease in the future, as they experience increased work-related stress. Partly because of the "wonder woman" myth, white-collar women are less likely to stop smoking than their male counterparts. Women must begin following a heart-healthy lifestyle in their early adult years, in preparation for the postmenopausal years when their risk-factor profile takes a serious turn for the worse.

MYTH 4. AGE

Younger people naturally like to believe that heart attacks occur only to the elderly. That gives them decades to wait before altering their unhealthy lifestyles. One visit to the cardiac care unit of a hospital would put an end to this myth. Many people, mostly males, have heart attacks in their 50's, 40's, even 30's. In most cases, you can avoid becoming an early heart-attack victim by taking the concept of risk factors seriously. One emergency medical care specialist says that when he's treating heart-attack victims under age 45, the first thing he does is look around for a pack of cigarettes.

MYTH 5. SUDDENNESS

Too many people believe that heart disease and heart attacks appear suddenly like a bolt of lightning. They blame an event such as an argument for "causing" the heart attack. This is rarely, if ever, accurate. Heart attacks are usually made possible by atherosclerosis of the coronary arteries, as the buildup of fatty deposits gradually restricts the flow of blood. After several decades, when the restriction is great enough, a heart attack occurs. True, a stressful event may immediately precede an attack — but without narrowed arteries or an otherwise compromised cardiovascular system, there would likely be no attack.

MYTH 6. TOO MUCH EXERCISE

This myth states that people with heart disease or many risk factors, should not exercise because it is too dangerous. If you fit this disease profile, you should obviously check with your physician prior to beginning any exercise program. But in most cases, your doctor will be extremely supportive; the notion that a sedentary life is a heart-healthy life was discarded decades ago. Remember Ike? His doctor prescribed golf — and not just riding in the cart.

MYTH 7. THE CURE

It would be nice if it were true that medication, angioplasty, and bypass surgery could "cure" heart disease. These treatments have dramatically improved the prognosis for many heart-disease patients. But they do not stop the disease process which resulted in the original blocked artery. Patients who have undergone one of these procedures must pay particular attention to their risk-factor profile.

MYTH 8. OVER THE HILL

Older adults sometimes believe that lifestyle changes are useless at their advanced age. They still smoke, eat foods high in saturated fat, drink many martinis, and refuse to exercise. Benefits of a heart-healthy lifestyle are not limited to just the young. Older adults enjoy improved breathing and vigor, the possibility that their doctors will decrease their medications, and an overall improved quality of life. Surely these benefits are worth working for.

HYPERTENSION AND YOUR HEART

We have all heard people say that they can't have hypertension because they don't feel tense. Hypertension is *not nervous tension*. As too many of you have come to know, it means high blood pressure — the pressure your heart exerts on your blood vessels.

Blood pressure varies according to the situation, time of day, and level of activity. There is even "white-coat hypertension" — blood pressure artificially elevated in the presence of a physician! You must have several blood pressure readings before a diagnosis of hypertension is firmly established.

Your blood pressure has two readings. The upper number is your *systolic* blood pressure — the pressure when your heart contracts; a systolic reading of 140 is at the upper limit of the *normal* range. The lower number is your *diastolic* blood pressure — the pressure while your heart is resting between beats; this figure should be 90 or less. *Ideal readings are lower — systolic pressure under 120 and diastolic in the 60's or 70's.* Even mildly-elevated blood pressure readings such as 150/94 signal an increased risk of heart attack or stroke. A sad fact is that almost half of all hypertensives are not even aware they have high blood pressure. They are walking around like ticking time bombs!

The causes of hypertension are not completely understood. It runs in families, but it is not clear whether this is because of genetics, or because family members are more likely to have similar lifestyles. Virtually all experts agree that a combination of genetics and lifestyle contributes to most cases of hypertension. Lifestyle factors include smoking, obesity, excessive sodium intake, lack of exercise, stress, too little potassium in the diet, and a need for calcium and magnesium boosted by vitamin D.

8 WAYS TO A HEALTHY HEART

(1) It is also likely that three specific vitamins will be of help to your heart. The evidence points to *vitamin E* as helping to raise HDL levels, and to protecting artery walls and the heart muscle. *Vitamin C* has been shown to decrease cholesterol levels and protect against blood clotting, while *B6* helps keep blood from becoming sticky and tending to clot.

(2) And don't forget the minerals; *calcium* to lower cholesterol levels, and *magnesium* for the efficient functioning of the heart muscle.

190

(3) If you are overweight, a return to normal weight will often return your blood pressure to normal.

(4) It is also important to reduce your sodium intake. Excess sodium causes your body to retain fluid, forcing the heart to work harder pumping the extra fluid. Potato chips, canned soups, canned vegetables, and frozen dinners are major sources of sodium. Read product labels; after awhile, your taste buds will tell you when something is too salty. Your physician may prescribe diuretics to decrease the fluid in your system and lighten your heart's work load. But medication should supplement dietary changes, not substitute for them.

(5) In addition, aerobic exercise lowers resting heart rate, and lets your heart function more efficiently.

(6) Learn to handle stress. Accept life's trials and tribulations with a shrug, or as a challenge. Learn to laugh away your troubles. Learn to handle them rather than letting them handle you. Your heart will appreciate it.

(7) For a heart-healthy diet, you need foods high in potassium — bananas, broccoli, potatoes with skins on, cantaloupe, raisins, and dates. Go to your health food store for calcium-magnesium tablets. And get plenty of vitamin D — from foods, capsules, or sunshine.

(8) A dosage of 325mg *every other day* — *one* common garden variety *aspirin* — has great health benefits, even for those who have already suffered a heart attack. One recent discovery is that an aspirin every other day can help prevent heart attacks. According to the *New England Journal of Medicine*, *aspirin*, or the prescription drug *Coumadin* can reduce by three-fold the risk of blood-clotting that can lead to strokes or heart attacks. The advantage of aspirin is that it doesn't have the side effects of *Coumadin* and is simpler and cheaper to obtain.

CIGARETTE SMOKING AND HEART DISEASE

One obvious effect of cigarette smoking is increased heart rate — an increase of 15 to 20 beats per minute! In addition, *irregular heartbeats* are more common in smokers. When your heart beats faster, it works harder, even in smokers who regularly participate in aerobic exercise. Smoking also increases blood pressure. This puts hypertensive smokers at double the risk for heart disease. Smoking increases clotting in veins and arteries; it adds poisonous carbon monoxide to the blood, and lowers HDL cholesterol — the "good" cholesterol that you were busy raising through your aerobic exercise program.

Using a substance that speeds heart rate, raises blood pressure, and decreases levels of HDL cholesterol is like playing *Russian Roulette*. If you pull the trigger enough times, your luck will eventually run out.

Even a one-pack-a-day smoker increases their heart-disease risk threefold. This risk is multiplied tremendously, if smokers have high blood pressure, diabetes, high cholesterol, or obesity. A smoker with two or three additional risk factors may have a thirty- or forty-fold increase in risk.

Even *second-hand smoke* can increase heart-disease risk by 30%. But if you stop smoking, your risk of heart disease *immediately* begins to decrease. After five nonsmoking years, most former smokers have heart-disease risks similar to lifelong *nonsmokers*. But don't keep postponing the start of your five-year plan — or you'll wake up in the hospital with no time left!

CHOLESTEROL AND YOUR HEART

Cholesterol is the health buzzword of the 1990's. This is a positive sign, but the danger is that some companies have launched unscrupulous advertising campaigns designed to cash in on the public's health-consciousness by putting "no cholesterol" on everything from cereal to cookies to pet food.

Cholesterol is a fatty substance which is manufactured by your body, and is necessary for normal health. It is a member of a class of fats called *lipids*. Three types of lipids can endanger your health —cholesterol, low-density lipoproteins (LDL), and triglycerides. Excessive amounts of any one of these can clog coronary arteries and restrict blood, requiring surgery or causing a heart attack.

According to the National Cholesterol Education Program, the *desirable level of cholesterol* and other lipids is *below* 200. Between 200 and 239 is on the borderline; over 240 is considered high. If your level is above 200, your physician may order blood tests for lipid profile on low-density lipoproteins (LDL), high-density lipoproteins (HDL) and triglycerides. *LDL levels* should be below 130, and *triglycerides* should be below 150. *HDL* (the "good guy") should be above 45. The ratio of your total cholesterol to your HDL level should not exceed 5 to 1. Thus a total cholesterol of 200 and an HDL level of 40 would barely be acceptable.

Some new research suggests that levels of *Apo B*, a protein found in LDL, may be the best predictor of heart disease in *women*, and levels of *Apo A-1* in HDL, the best predictor for *men*. Testing for these components is relatively inexpensive, so in a few years, we may have an even more accurate predictor of heart-disease risk.

Why is LDL bad, while HDL is good? LDL carries cholesterol to your *cells* where it is stored, resulting in higher cholesterol levels; HDL carries it to your *liver* where it is eventually excreted, resulting in lower cholesterol.

Blood cholesterol level depends on a combination of hereditary and lifestyle factors. In the worst genetic cases, a person may have familial *hypercholesterolemia* in which cholesterol will reach extremely dangerous levels at a very young age regardless of diet. While this is a rare condition, it makes premature heart disease extremely likely if the condition is not detected. This is why young children should have their cholesterol levels checked if there is a history of premature heart disease or high cholesterol levels in the family.

For 99% of people with high cholesterol levels, diet is the major culprit. Cholesterol is found in animal products such as meat, eggs, butter, and cheese. It is not found in grain, fruit, vegetables or vegetable oils, because plants do not produce cholesterol. Thus it is absurd to place "no cholesterol" labels on grain products such as cereals. An even larger contributor to blood cholesterol is *saturated fat* — fats which are solid or semi-solid at room temperature. Be wary of "hydrogenated" and "partially hydrogenated" oils; these indicate saturated fat, and many "no cholesterol" products are loaded with it.

If your cholesterol level is elevated, your doctor will probably recommend diet and exercise. *Exercise helps elevate your beneficial HDL cholesterol*, while decreasing weight to lower total cholesterol. Limit fat to 15-20% of your daily calories. *Use monounsaturated olive oil and polyunsaturated corn oil, soybean oil, sunflower oil, or that best cholesterol-buster, canola oil, which is rich in Omega-3.*

A 1% drop in cholesterol leads to a 2% decrease in heart disease risk. Cholesterol level is a more important consideration for those with other risk factors, so a slightly elevated cholesterol level is far more significant if you are a hypertensive smoker.

OBESITY AND HEART DISEASE

Society and the workplace discriminate against the obese, but it is the cardiovascular system which truly discriminates — it functions efficiently for more years in normal weight people than in obese people. Extra body fat requires the heart to work harder, pumping blood through more body mass.

Obese people often suffer from hypertension and high cholesterol levels, because obesity itself raises cholesterol, and most obese people eat too much fatty food. Obesity also increases the risk of Type II or adult-onset diabetes, which is a serious risk factor in heart disease. Finally, obese people are less likely to exercise, so they miss the heart-healthy benefits of an aerobic exercise program.

EXERCISE AND HEART DISEASE

The effects of a regular program of aerobic exercise are directly opposite those of cigarette smoking. Smoking increases resting heart rate; aerobic exercise decreases it, and decreases the work load on your heart. Cigarette smoking increases blood pressure;

and aerobic exercise lowers it, making the heart operate more efficiently. And cigarette smoking lowers levels of HDL or good cholesterol; but aerobic exercise increases HDL.

Exercise helps you handle stress, and most importantly, exercise actually strengthens your heart muscle. A sedentary lifestyle is one of the leading risk factors for the development of heart disease.

PERSONALITY, STRESS, AND HEART DISEASE

As discussed earlier, the anger or hostility associated with Type A behavior increases the risk of heart disease. Frequent outbursts of anger take a toll on your cardiovascular system. Other Type A characteristics such as *ambition* and *workaholism* do *not* appear to pose independent threats to your health.

Two types of anger create risk for heart disease: the *constant anger* of the person who finds it hard to control tantrums, who lashes out at everyone, turning red in the face, appearing ready to pop an artery. The second type is *internalized anger*, the source of constant frustration, depression, anxiety. Both types cause the rapid heart rate, increased blood pressure, and other physical changes associated with the fight-

or-flight response. Both groups need to alter their responses to situations, through exercise and relaxation techniques.

Another type of stress which is of great concern is the weakening of the immune systems in people who have suffered a loss — the death of a loved one, the loss of a job or home. Individuals in these situations should use the stress reduction techniques discussed in this book, and for awhile, try to avoid significant changes in their lives which could add stress.

QUIZ: WHAT IS YOUR RISK OF DEVELOPING HEART DISEASE?

Obviously, this quiz cannot take into account every detail of your particular case. Only your doctor can do that. But a high score on this quiz is a strong suggestion that you should visit a doctor.

1. Your systolic (first or higher number) blood pressure is usually
   - a. below 120 (1 point)
   - b. 120-139 (2 points)
   - c. 140-159 (5 points)
   - d. 160-199 (10 points)
   - e. over 200 (20 points)

2. Your diastolic (second or lower number) blood pressure is usually
     a. below 80   (1 point)
     b. 80-89   (2 points)
     c. 90-99   (5 points)
     d. 100-109   (10 points)
     e. over 110   (20 points)

3. Your cholesterol level is
     a. below 200 (1 point)
     b. 200-219   (2 points)
     c. 220-239   (5 points)
     d. 240-279   (10 points)
     e. over 280   (20 points)

4. Your LDL cholesterol is
     a. below 130 (1 point)
     b. 130-145   (2 points)
     c. 145-159   (5 points)
     d. 160-189   (10 points)
     e. over 190   (20 points)

5. Which statement is true?
     a. Never smoked (1 point)
     b. Quit smoking more than 5 years ago (2 points)
     c. Quit smoking more than 1 year ago (5 points)

d. Quit smoking less than 1 year ago
(10 points)

e. Currently smoke (20 points)

6. Which statement is true?

a. Do not smoke (1 point)

b. Smoke less than 1/2 pack per day
(2 points)

c. Smoke 1/2 to 1 pack per day
(5 points)

d. Smoke 1 to 2 packs per day
(10 points)

e. Smoke more than 2 packs per day
(20 points)

7. Which statement is true?

a. Male under 45 or woman under
55 (1 point)

b. Male under 55 or woman under
65 (2 points)

c. Male under 65 or woman over 65
(5 points)

d. Male over 65 (10 points)

8. Do you currently have diabetes?

a. No (1 point)

b. Developed diabetes after age 65
(5 points)

c. Developed diabetes after age 55
(10 points)
d. Developed diabetes before age 55
(20 points)

9. Which describes you best?
a. Vigorous exercise 3-6 times per
week (1 point)
b. Moderate exercise 3-6 times per
week (2 points)
c. Moderate or vigorous exercise 2
times per week (5 points)
d. Exercise less than 2 times per week
(10 points)
e. Rarely or never exercise (20 points)

10. You would describe yourself as
a. Rarely feeling stressed (1 point)
b. Moderately stressed at home or
work (2 points)
c. Moderately stressed at home and
at work (5 points)
d. Extremely stressed at home or at
work (10 points)
e. Extremely stressed at home and at
work (20 points)

11. Which of the following statements is true?

a. Both of your parents lived past age 75 and did not suffer a stroke or heart attack (1 point)

b. Both of your parents lived past age 75 or did not suffer a stroke or heart attack before age 75 (2 points)

c. One or both of your parents had a stroke or heart attack before age 75 (3 points)

d. One or both of your parents had a stroke or heart attack before age 65 (5 points)

e. One or both of your parents had a stroke or heart attack before age 55 (10 points)

f. One or both of your parents had a stroke or heart attack before age 45 (20 points)

SCORE ANALYSIS

11-16 —EXTREMELY LOW RISK - You are doing the right things and should keep it up.

17-30 —LOW RISK - While there is some room for improvement, you are doing a good job in protecting yourself from heart disease.

203

31-40 —MILD RISK - While you are doing better than most people, you should check your answers for areas where improvement is needed.

41-50 —MODERATE RISK - Your profile merits attention. There are several problem areas which should be addressed.

51-75 —HIGH RISK - Now is a good time to address your risk profile. There are a number of problem areas.

76-100 —VERY HIGH RISK - Your situation merits attention by your family physician.

101 OR ABOVE —EXTREME RISK - Your situation merits immediate attention by your family physician.

CHAPTER 11

REDUCING YOUR RISK OF CANCER

In a Cancer Prevention Awareness Survey conducted in 1983 by the National Cancer Institute
(NCI), the director, Dr. Vincent De Vita, reported:

"Only 38% of the population expressed
the belief that cancer risk is related to lifestyle.
And when asked if they had ever talked to a
doctor about ways to reduce their chances of
getting cancer, almost 86% said 'no.' But
when asked how likely they would be to follow a doctor's advice on ways to reduce can-

cer risk, almost two-thirds said they would be 'very likely.'

"I think there is a dual message to be drawn from this survey. The first is that our patients need to understand that lifestyle choices are indeed connected to cancer and that individuals have the opportunity and the power to reduce their cancer risks. The second message is that we physicians have credibility with our patients, and they do listen to us, but we are missing the boat if we do not make active attempts to counsel patients about ways they can reduce their cancer risks...

"To me, the opportunity to prevent cancer is one of the most exciting challenges ever. It is an opportunity that we can all share."

Scientists generally agree that about 80% of cancer cases are tied to the way people live — the foods they eat, the work they do, smoking, too much sun. Of course some factors, like your work environment, are harder to control; but others are easy, like eating the proper foods, and not smoking.

SMOKING AND CANCER

The most important thing you can do to avoid getting cancer is to *avoid first-and second-hand tobacco smoke*. Although other cancers are diagnosed more — prostate cancer in men, breast and colon or rectal cancer in women — lung cancer kills more men and women. Smoking causes 30% of all cancer deaths, and those who smoke have a ten-times greater chance of getting cancer than those who don't.

People who smoke cigars and pipes are less likely to develop lung cancer if they don't inhale, but are at serious risk for cancers of the mouth, tongue, and throat. Use of snuff and chewing tobacco can lead to cancer of the mouth. The message is clear — *stay away from all tobacco!*

In addition, *smoking ages you drastically*. It shrinks the fine capillaries, causing the skin to wrinkle years too early, and it cuts off the blood supply to the skin, causing a grey pallor. Health and beauty — they go together.

DIET AND CANCER

Certain foods and nutrients are associated with cancer. A high intake of fat is a risk factor for cancer

Vibrant Health

of the colon, breasts, prostate, stomach, kidneys, gall bladder, and the lining of the uterus. A twelve-year study conducted by the American Cancer Society found a marked *increase of these cancers in obese people.*

Keep your intake of all fats low — both saturated and unsaturated fats. Choose lean red meats, fish, and white-meat poultry. Trim fat from steaks, roasts, and chops before cooking; skin poultry before cooking. Try broiling, roasting, or baking meats and fish, or simmering them in their own juices — anything but frying them. Limit your use of butter, margarine, cream, shortening, and even vegetable oils. Avoid hidden fats in salad dressings and especially snack foods like potato chips. Choose skim or low-fat milk, low-fat cheeses and dairy desserts. Choose fruit instead of high-fat desserts, and ice milk instead of ice cream.

Other foods help reduce your cancer risk. The three most important *antioxidants* (which stop tumor formation) are *vitamins C and E*, and the trace mineral *selenium.* Eat fresh fruits, especially those high in vitamins A and C — oranges, grapefruit, nectarines, peaches, cantaloupe, honeydew melons, and all berries. In addition, a daily vitamin-C-500mg. supplement is a wise course of action for anyone to help prevent cancer.

Vitamin E is found in whole grains, wheat germ, sunflower seeds and vegetable oils. If you eat white bread, change to whole-grain breads. And take a vitamin-E supplement, as well as selenium.

The best cancer fighter of all may be *vitamin A*. The natural coloring agent in orange and yellow fruits and vegetables, and in dark green leafy vegetables is called *beta-carotene*, which is converted in the body to vitamin A. Diets low in vitamin A have been linked to cancers of the prostrate, cervix, skin, bladder, colon, larynx, and lung. Supplements of beta-carotene and vitamin A are readily available.

One important element in the fight against cancer is *garlic*, which seems to reduce the formation of cancer-causing substances in the stomach. Non-odorous capsules are available.

Dietary *fiber*, the partially nondigestible material in plant cells, helps move food quickly through the intestines and out of the body. It helps prevent constipation, and promotes a healthy digestive tract. Foods high in fiber protect against some cancers, particularly colorectal. Diets high in fat increase risk for these cancers.

To get enough fiber, eat several servings of fresh fruits and vegetables, peas and beans, breads and cereals from whole grains, daily. Eating large amounts of these fiber-rich goods, known as *complex carbohydrates*, won't make you gain weight, particularly if you're cutting down on fat.

Eliminate all salt-cured, pickled, and smoked foods. Smoked ham or salt pork carry a double negative whammy—high fat combined with the way they are processed. Avoid even smoked fish or smoked anything. That means cutting down on the summer barbecues.

Many studies have concluded that moderate alcohol use (one or two drinks per day) does *no harm* — although there is mounting evidence that *women who have as few as three drinks per week are at increased risk for breast cancer.* If you are a woman already at risk for breast cancer (obese, mother or sister with breast cancer, no children or first pregnancy after age 30) drinking should be minimal or avoided completely. And no amount of alcohol is advisable during pregnancy.

Heavy drinking in men or women can cause cancers of the mouth, throat, esophagus, and liver.

Smokers who drink have an even higher risk of getting cancers of the mouth and esophagus.

EXERCISE AND CANCER

Exercise not only prevents heart attacks, it also seems to prevent cancer. As far back as 1922, Ivar Sivertsen and A.W. Dahlstrom published a report in *The Journal of Cancer Research* showing that, "The death rate among males actively engaged in a gainful occupation is inversely proportional to the degree of muscular activity necessary for that occupation." (Females weren't studied "because of the difficulty in estimating the amount of muscular activity relative to occupations of this sex.")

In 1961, S.A. Hoffman and others at Jefferson Medical College in Philadelphia compared tumor growth in rats vigorously exercised to those confined or not exercised. "In each instance the weight of the tumor in the control group significantly exceeded that in the exercised group. In several instances there was complete tumor regression in the exercised animals." Further experiments indicate that when a muscle is exercised to fatigue, it apparently produces a substance that limits the activity of cancerous tumors. So we have ample evidence that *exercise helps prevent cancer*, even if we don't know precisely why.

211

ENVIRONMENTAL AND OTHER FACTORS
SUNLIGHT

Long exposure to sunlight has been linked to skin cancer. The sun's ultraviolet (UV) rays which harm the skin are strongest and the risk is greatest from 11 a.m. to 2 p.m. during the summer. Fair-skinned, and especially freckled, people are at a greater risk than dark-skinned people, because the dark pigment called *melanin* helps block some of the sun's damaging rays. The harm from over-exposure to sunlight is never fully repaired, even after the suntan or sunburn fades away. Besides that, the sun ages and wrinkles the skin drastically.

You can protect yourself by wearing long-sleeved shirts, long pants, and a broad-brimmed hat, and by using sunscreens. A number 15 on the label means most the sun's UV rays will be blocked out. Any number higher than that has not proved any more effective. Not even a beach umbrella gives full protection, since you receive dangerous reflected sun rays from off the sand.

X-RAYS

Large doses of radiation are known to cause cancer. Although you are exposed to very little radiation in a single X-ray, getting many X-rays over a long period does increase your cancer risk. Discuss each X-ray with your doctor or dentist; take only those X-rays that are necessary; and ask that X-ray shields be used to protect other parts of your body.

ESTROGEN

Studies seemed to show, in the 1970's, that women who took large doses of estrogen for menopause symptoms had six to seven times the risk of developing endometrial cancer than women who did not take estrogen. Today, estrogen is carefully given with a form of progesterone to balance it — and this seems to nullify any risk of uterine cancer. In fact, some gynecologists now strongly recommend this balanced hormone to menopausal and postmenopausal women, to prevent osteoporosis and lessen their risk of heart attack and stroke. One negative factor with estrogen-replacement therapy is a slight increase in risk for breast cancer (more of a concern for women with a family history of breast cancer). Smoking diminishes the benefits of this treatment.

Women on estrogen therapy and those using birth-control pills should examine their breasts regularly, and get regular mammograms and *Pap* tests. There is no conclusive evidence that cancer is caused by any of the birth-control pills now on the market, but the risk of breast and cervical cancer might be higher in some individuals. On the other hand, there is some evidence that pill-users may have a lower risk of cancers of the uterine lining and ovary.

ON-THE-JOB EXPOSURE

Three kinds of workplace substances increase cancer risks: *chemicals, metals,* and *dusts or fibers.* Only a small number of agents in these groups actually cause cancer — most often in combination with another workplace carcinogen, or with cigarette smoke. *Asbestos* fibers create an especially high risk of lung disease, and the risk is even higher for workers who smoke. Some scientists suggest that the main carcinogen in the workplace is the *cigarette!*

Labor unions, industry, and regulatory agencies, such as OSHA, have developed health and safety measures for the workplace. These measures should be known and followed.

BUMPS, BRUISES, OR OTHER INJURIES

That bump you got playing basketball won't cause cancer, but sometimes, treatment for an injury leads the doctor to find a cancer that had gone undetected.

Irritants over a long period of time, however, (such as snuff against the gums) can cause cancer.

OTHER FACTORS

We might begin to believe that anything can cause cancer if the dose is high enough. High doses of many chemicals are toxic, but they will not cause cancer. *Toxicity*, causing loss of hair or weight, various organ malfunctions, or even death, should not be confused with carcinogenesis.

No one knows for sure how a normal cell becomes a cancer cell, but scientists agree that people get cancer mainly through repeated or long-term contact with one or more cancer-causing agents called *carcinogens*. Cancers develop slowly, usually appearing 5 to 40 years after exposure to a cancer-causing agent. This long latent period is one reason why it is so difficult to identify the causes of human cancer. Lung cancer, for example, may not appear until 30 years after exposure to second-hand tobacco smoke, or asbestos.

CHAPTER 12

HOW LONG WILL YOU LIVE?

If there is one question which all of you would like us to answer, it is probably, "How long am I going to live?" Obviously, there is no definitive answer for any of us. In a world beset by homicides, drunk drivers, and natural disasters, we can't even be sure that we will live to see the sun rise tomorrow. But given the role of luck in longevity, why do you do things that you know are going to cut down the odds of being lucky enough to live a long healthy, life?

THE WALLINGFORD LONGEVITY TEST

This test is not appropriate if you are elderly, have a major illness, or have an unusual family history of a disease. If none of these are the case for you, give the test a try and see how you are doing in your effort to live to see your children enjoy their retirement.

Each person begins the test with 75 years. All additional numbers are either added to or subtracted from 75. Obviously, a key goal is to have more additions than subtractions.

CHOLESTEROL

Total Cholesterol Level

Below 175 .... +2
176-200 .... +1
201-240 .... -1
241-280 .... -2
281-320 .... -4
Over 320 .... -6

BLOOD PRESSURE

SYSTOLIC
(First or Higher Number)

Below 120 .... +2
121-140 .... +1
141-160 .... -1
161-180 .... -2
181-200 .... -3
Over 200 .... -4

DIASTOLIC
(Second or Lower Number)

Below 70 .... +2
71- 80 .... +1
81- 90 0
91-100 .... -1
101-110 .... -2
111-120 .... -3
Over 120 .... -4

HDL CHOLESTEROL

Over 60 .... +2
51-59 .... +1
41-50 0
31-40 .... -1
26-30 .... -3
Below 26 .... -5

FAMILY HISTORY
PART I

Average age at death of your
four grandparents

Over 80 .... +2
75-79 .... +1
70-74 0
60-69 .... -2
50-59 .... -4
Below 50 .... -6

(Do not count grandparents who died as a result of
suicide, homicide, accidental death, drug overdose,
or other unnatural causes.)

FAMILY HISTORY
Part II

Both parents free of both cancer
and heart disease at age 70 .... +2

One parent free of both cancer and
heart disease at age 70, and other
parent free of these diseases at age 60 +1

Both parents free of cancer
and heart disease at age 60 0

One parent developed cancer
or heart disease in his/her 50's .... -1

Both parents developed cancer
or heart disease in their 50's .... -3

One parent developed cancer
or heart disease prior to age 50 .... -4

Both parents developed cancer
or heart disease prior to age 50 .... -6

Vibrant Health

WEIGHT

Normal .... +2
 0-10 pounds overweight .... -1
11-20 pounds overweight.............. -2
21-30 pounds overweight .... -3
31-40 pounds overweight .... -4
41-60 pounds overweight .... -5
More than 60 pounds overweight .. -7

EXERCISE

30 minutes or more of moderate
exercise at least 5 times per week +3

30 minutes or more of moderate
exercise 3 or 4 times per week ..... +2

30 minutes or more of moderate
exercise 2 times per week .... +1

No regular aerobic exercise
program .... -3

ALCOHOL

0-2 drinks per week .... +2
3-7 drinks per week 0
8-14 drinks per week .... -1
15-21 drinks per week .... -2
22-28 drinks per week .... -4
At least 8 drinks per week and
smoke cigarettes .... -7

TOBACCO
(choose all that apply)

Never smoked .... +3
Quit smoking at least five years ago .... +2
Quit smoking less than five years ago 0
Currently smoke, but less than one pack of
cigarettes a day .... -1
Currently smoke approximately one pack of
cigarettes a day .... -3
Currently smoke approximately two packs of
cigarettes a day .... -5
Currently smoke approximately three
packs of cigarettes a day .... -7
Have smoked for 25 years or more .... -3

223

NUTRITION
(choose all that apply)

Consistently eat a well-balanced diet ...... +2
Inconsistent eating habits .... -2
Eat 3 meals per day .... +1
Skip meals .... -1
Eat a daily breakfast high in
complex carbohydrates and fiber .... +2
Either skip or eat a high
fat breakfast .... -2
Eat fish and poultry rather
than red meat .... +2
Eat red meat rather than
fish or poultry .... -2
Eat at least 7 servings of
vegetables weekly .... +1
Eat at least 7 servings of fruit weekly ...... +1
Eat a low fat diet .... +2
Eat a high fat diet .... -2
Avoid fried foods .... +1
Frequently eat fried foods .... -1

(If your score in the nutrition section is more than +5 or less than –5, use +5 or –5 in your calculations rather than the more extreme number.)

STRESS
(choose all that apply)

Almost always relaxed .... +2
Frequently angry .... -3
Often tense .... -1
Usually happy .... +1
Often depressed .... -1
Laugh often .... +1
Rarely laugh .... -1
Feel good about yourself.............. +1
Low self worth .... -1
Financial problems .... -1
Financially stable .... +1
Like your job .... +1
Hate your job .... -1
Several good friends .... +1
Have no good friends .... -1
Happy family life........................... +1
Unhappy family life....................... -1

(If your score in the stress section is more than +5 or less than –5, use +5 or –5 in your calculations rather than the more extreme number.

SEX

Male.. -3

Female .... +3

If your total score is a high number, it looks like your life is heading in the right direction. If the number is very low, it may be time to examine some of your behaviors such as smoking and drinking excessively, which can have an adverse effect on your health. Look back at your minuses. Can you change these behaviors? Pick one and work on it.

CONCLUSION

Congratulations! You have just completed *Vibrant Health*. What we have tried to do in this book is to provide you with information to allow you to make healthy choices in your life. However, reading this book is only the first step on your journey to better living. *Implementation is the key.* You must ask yourself if you are truly interested, motivated, even excited by reading about the accomplishments of others and the possibilities for yourself.

Our main purpose is not to show you how to lose weight, although if you need to, you probably will if you incorporate even a few of the *Vibrant Health* changes in your life.

Our main purpose is to show you how to enjoy a healthier, happier life now, and for as long as you live. That is the real message to be found in *Vibrant Health*. It is a message of quality and vitality of life.

Through proper nutrition, exercise, and stress reduction, you can enjoy life to the fullest. You can begin to see that *your* choices, *your* behaviors, determine what happens to you — not 100% of the time but most of the time. Don't fall into the trap of believing that because you can't control everything that you control nothing. Remember the serenity prayer and dedicate the rest of your life to achieving a greater level of *Vibrant Health*.

Dr. Clifford Stewart, Ph.D.

Clifford Stewart holds a Ph.D. in psychology, has published over 50 publications and papers which include a book on cancer, *Cancer: Prevention, Detection, Causes, Treatment*, two encyclopedia articles, and numerous publications in professional journals.

He has studied and taught various aspects of health care over a period of 25 years. Dr. Stewart has taught health care delivery at Claremont Graduate School (CA), guest-lectured at the School of Allied Health Professions, Loma Linda University (CA), piloted a cancer screening program for the American Cancer Society, and currently serves on the Board of Health for the City of Chester, and teaches behavioral medicine at Widener University (PA).

Dr. Stewart has helped establish Health Maintenance Organizations in California and New York, and has served on the boards of these organizations. He is active in research in biofeedback, and currently is president of the Pennsylvania Society of Behavioral Medicine and Biofeedback.

Dr. Lawrence A. Fehr, Ph.D.

Lawrence A. Fehr received his M.A. degree in psychology from Fairleigh Dickinson University in 1974 and his Ph.D. in psychology from the University of Cincinnati in 1977. He has served on the faculty of Lehigh University, and is currently an Associate Professor of Psychology at Widener University in Chester, Pennsylvania.

During the last 15 years, Dr. Fehr has been the author of over 80 books, including *Introduction to Personality, Theories of Stress*, articles, and papers concerning the importance and nature of stress reduction, wellness, anxiety, aggression, self-esteem and other related topics. His work has been published in numerous professional periodicals including the *American Psychologist, Journal of Personality Assessment, Journal of Genetic Psychology, Journal of Youth and Adolescence, Merrill-Palmer Quarterly, and Human Development*. In addition, he has presented countless lectures and workshops on these topics to professional and popular audiences throughout the United States and Canada.

Dr. Fehr has been active in many notable organizations including the Eastern Psychological Association, Association for Management, and the Society for Personality Assessment. He also is a member and serves on the executive board of the National Social Science Association.

Being a believer in the importance of proper nutrition, stress reduction, and a regular program of aerobic exercise for many years, he follows his own advice by adhering to a nutritional program which is extremely low in fat and high in complex carbohydrates. In addition, he can be found on either his treadmill or stationary bicycle during six hour-long session per week.

230

GLOSSARY

adrenaline - a secretion of the adrenal glands which, when released into the bloodstream, causes heightened emotional levels and increased strength.

aerobic exercise - continuous activity over a period of time involving the large muscle groups. It results in increased heart rate and an increased demand on the cardiovascular system. Examples include brisk walking, rowing, swimming, cycling, and jogging.

anaerobic exercise - intense muscular activity that occurs in relatively short bursts of effort. Examples include weight lifting and sprinting.

android obesity - condition in which the majority of excess weight is located above the waist. This type of obesity is associated with increased risk of heart disease and is most commonly found in males.

angioplasty - procedure in which a partially blocked coronary artery is reopened through the use of a balloon tipped catheter.

anorexia nervosa - eating disorder in which people reduce their weight to unsafe levels. In spite of the weight loss, they continue to perceive themselves as fat. The condition often begins during adolescence and is more common in females than in males.

autogenic training - a relaxation technique that emphasizes imagery and self-suggestion.

blood pressure - the pressure your heart exerts on your blood vessels.

biofeedback - getting objective information about the state of one's body and its functioning. Also, a method of training used in learning to control one's physiological processes.

body fat percentage - the percentage of a person's total body weight which is fat. This is a better method of determining obesity than pounds noted on a scale.

bypass surgery - surgical procedure actually called *coronary artery bypass graft surgery* in which one or more coronary arteries which are severely blocked are "bypassed" at the point of blockage through the use of an artery or vein from another part of the body.

calorie - a measure of the energy value of foods. It is technically the amount of heat required to raise the temperature of one kilogram of water 1 degree centigrade.

carbohydrates - any of a group of compounds containing carbon combined with hydrogen and oxygen. It includes simple sugars as well as starches.

cardiac arrhythmia - abnormalities in the rhythm of the heartbeat. The severity of the problem varies dramatically from harmless and occasional premature contractions to other life-threatening irregularities.

cardiovascular disease - the technical term for heart disease.

cholesterol - an odorless fatty substance manufactured by your body. Also found in animal products (meat, cheese, eggs, etc.). It is a member of a class of fats called *lipids*.

complex carbohydrates - the type of carbohydrates found in large quantities in fruits, vegetables and grains. They should represent the majority of your daily intake of calories.

cool-down - gradual decrease of effort at the end of an exercise program. It enables your heart to return slowly to its resting rate and to avoid post-exercise soreness. Stretching is part of that process.

cross-training - alternating activities such as brisk walking, swimming, and rowing during your weekly workouts. This enables you to avoid boredom and also to work different muscle groups.

carbon monoxide - a colorless, odorless, poisonous gas contained in cigarette smoke. While smoking, it replaces some of the oxygen in your blood.

diabetes - a disease of metabolism characterized by the body's inability to use sugar.

diastolic blood pressure - this is the second or lower number in your blood pressure reading. It is the pressure that exists as your heart readies itself or rests up in preparation for its next beat.

dietary cholesterol - cholesterol found in foods. It is contained only in animal products such as meat, butter, and cheese.

diet pills - these are pills taken in place of or in conjunction with a specified program of nutrition. The pills usually are either diuretics which decrease fluids in the body or stimulants designed to increase one's metabolic rate.

diuretics - drugs which decrease the fluids in the body and which decrease the effort which the heart must exert in order to perform its pumping action. These are the most widely prescribed medications for hypertension.

endorphins - substances produced by the body, similar in effect to opium, and important in internal pain regulation.

estrogen - one of several hormones produced mainly by the ovary.

external locus of control - a belief that the rewards in your life are determined by factors beyond your control such as luck, fate, or other people.

fad diet - a diet which focuses on a specific food, food group, food supplement or is in some other way nutritionally deficient.

familial hypercholesterolemia - an inherited condition in which a person may have a dangerously high cholesterol level in the absence of inappropriate and unhealthy eating habits.

fast - a partial or total abstinence from food. This approach to weight loss is extremely dangerous when taken to extremes.

fat - any of a class of yellowish to white greasy, solid, or liquid substances found in plant and animal tissues. All oils are 100% fat.

fiber - this is found exclusively in plant foods. It is the part of the plant that is not broken down in the intestines in the process of digestion.

fight or flight - a syndrome accompanying activation of the sympathetic nervous system, resulting in increased readiness to fight or to run.

general adaptation syndrome - a three-stage process (alarm, resistance, exhaustion) describing the activities of the body under stress.

gynoid obesity - a condition in which the majority of excess weight is located below the waist. This condition is not associated with an increased risk of heart disease and is usually found in women.

hardiness - a concept used to describe the ability to maintain health during stressful periods.

HDL - high density lipoproteins. This is the good cholesterol which carries cholesterol to the liver where it is eventually excreted from the body.

heart attack - takes place when the blood supply to the heart is cut off by the complete blockage of one or more coronary arteries.

heart disease - a disease related to the heart. It commonly involves coronary artery disease in which atherosclerosis has taken place. This involves the buildup of deposits inside an artery which can partially or totally block blood flow.

heart rate - the number of heart beats which occur in one minute.

hydrogenated oils - oils in which processing has resulted in increased hardening or saturation. This renders the oil less desirable from a health perspective because of the increased likelihood that it will raise one's cholesterol level.

hypertension - the technical term for high blood pressure. It is not nervous tension.

incontinence - the inability to control excretory functions.

insoluble fiber - this speeds up the movement of food through the intestines. This enables a person's bowel movements to be regular. It is found in kidney beans, peas, and whole-wheat products.

internal locus of control - the belief that you control the events in your life.

interval training - alternating the intensity and duration of exercise both within and across workouts.

junk food - term often used for snack foods and fast food meals. There is a wide range of nutritional desirability within this category. For example, hot air popcorn is a healthy alternative to potato chips.

LDL - this is the bad cholesterol which carries cholesterol to the cells where it is stored.

liquid diet - a diet in which most or all of the meals do not contain solid food. Examples include *Optifast®* which is a medically supervised "all liquid" diet and *Ultra Slim Fast®* which is an over-the-counter product designed to be used in place of breakfast and lunch on a daily basis.

locus of control - your belief concerning what or who determines the rewards in your life.

mantra - in meditation, a word or phrase or sound thought of or uttered repeatedly and used as a target of complete concentration.

maximal heart rate - this is defined as 220 heart beats minus your age. It is used in the calculation of your target heart rate for exercise.

meditation - a process involving relaxation, slow, natural breathing, and the use of a mantra, with the objective being to clear the mind of stressful thoughts.

metabolic rate - the rate at which your body uses energy.

monounsaturated fat - fats which are liquid at room temperature and which are less complex than polyunsaturated fats. Olive oil and canola oil are heavy in monounsaturated fat. A part of a good diet.

multiple personality disorder - (MPD) two or more personalities in the same individual, any one of which may take control of the person's behavior.

myxedema - a condition involving severe deficiency of thyroid hormone, characterized by low body temperature, muscle weakness, and decreased mental functioning.

obesity - an extreme overweight condition often defined as being 25% overweight. A more appropriate approach is to focus on a person's percentage of body fat.

parasympathetic nervous system - that portion of the autonomic nervous system concerned with calming or reducing arousal.

personality - the complex of behaviors and underlying characteristics that distinguish one individual from another.

polyunsaturated fat - fats which are liquid at room temperature. These are found in the seeds of plants and are more complex than monounsaturated fats. Corn oil, safflower oil, soybean oil, and sunflower oil are high in polyunsaturated fat.

protein - a class of complex nitrogenous compounds originally found in plants and needed for human metabolism. Fish, skinless poultry, and low-fat dairy products are excellent sources of protein.

Raynaud's Disease - a condition characterized by seriously decreased blood circulation in the hands and feet, triggered by cold temperatures or by emotional stress.

resting heart rate - the number of times your heart beats in one minute while you are at rest. A good time to measure this rate is shortly after waking in the morning.

saturated fat - fats which are solid or semi-solid at room temperature. Coconut oil and palm oil are examples of highly saturated fats. Not recommended.

simple carbohydrates - the term for the simple sugars found in food. This type of carbohydrates provide "empty" calories and are associated with weight gain.

soluble fiber - this is fiber which slows down the movement of food through the intestines. This type of fiber seems to be useful in lowering blood cholesterol. It is found in oat bran, broccoli, apples, and pinto beans.

stress - a condition that occurs when a person must adapt to demands, as when an environmental event threatens them.

sympathetic nervous system - that part of the autonomic nervous system responsible for arousing or mobilizing the body for action.

systematic desensitization - a technique for alleviating anxiety involving progressive muscle relaxation training. Relaxation is then practiced while imagining or being exposed to anxiety-inducing situations.

systolic blood pressure - the first or upper number in a blood pressure reading. This is the amount of pressure which exists when the heart contracts.

target heart rate - this is determined by calculating 60 to 85% of the maximal heart rate. This is the rate at which most aerobic exercise should take place in order to derive maximum benefit.

triglycerides - a natural body fat found in the bloodstream. They are actually three fatty-acid chains attached to a glycerol molecule. Low triglyceride levels are desirable in our efforts to prevent heart disease.

Type A personality - displays extremely competitive, hostile, time-urgent behaviors; at their maximum when exposed to uncontrollable stress.

Type B personality - relative lack of Type A characteristics; a more relaxed style of coping.

type I diabetes - insulin dependent diabetes.

type II diabetes - non-insulin dependent diabetes.

warm up - the preparation of the body for vigorous aerobic exercise through a program of stretching and gradual increase in the intensity of the aerobic exercise.

white-coat hypertension - high blood pressure readings which occur when taken by the physician in his/her office but which are not duplicated in the home, work, or other environments.

yo-yo syndrome - the phenomenon in which repeated dieting alternated with over eating results in a repeated pattern of weight fluctuation. The loss of weight becomes more difficult with each repetition of the pattern.

BIBLIOGRAPHY AND RECOMMENDED READINGS

American Heart Association. (1973). *The American Heart Association Cookbook.* New York: Ballantine Books.

Anderson, T. (1980). *Stretching.* California: Shelter Publications.

Bennett, C. M., & Newport, C. (1987). *Control Your High Blood Pressure Cookbook.* New York: Doubleday & Co.

Benson, H. (1975). *The Relaxation Response.* New York: William Morrow & Company.

Benson, H., & Proctor, W. (1984). *Beyond the Relaxation Response: How to Harness the Healing Power of Your Personal Beliefs.* New York: Times Books.

Bielinski, R., Schutz, Y., & Jequier, E. (1985). "Energy metabolism in the post-exercise recovery in man 1,2." *American Journal of Clinical Nutrition, 42,* 69-82.

Bricklin, M. (1983). *The Practical Encyclopedia of Natural Healing.* Emmaus, PA: Rodale Press.

Brody, J. (1981). *Jane Brody's Nutrition Book.* New York: W. W. Norton.

Brody, J. (1985). *Jane Brody's Good Food Book.* New York: W. W. Norton & Co.

Brownell, K. D., and Foreyt, J. (1986). *Handbook of Eating Disorders.* New York: Basic Books.

Cash, T. F., Winstead, B. A., and Janda, L. H. (1986). "The great American shape-up." *Psychology Today, 20,* 4, 30-37.

241

Castelli, W. P., Doyle, J. T., & Gordon, T. (1977). "HDL cholesterol and other lipids in coronary heart disease." *Circulation,* 55, 767-772.

Castelli, W. P., Garrison, R., Wilson, P., Abbott, R., Kalousdian, S., & Kannel, W. (1986). "Incidence of coronary heart disease and lipoprotein cholesterol levels: the Framingham study." *Journal of the American Medical Association,* 256, 2835-2838.

Connor, S. L., & Connor, W. E. (1986). *The New American Diet.* New York: Simon & Schuster.

Cooper, K. H. (1988). *Controlling Cholesterol.* New York: Bantam Books.

Cottier, C., Shapiro, K., & Julius, S. (1984). "Treatment of mild hypertension with progressive muscle relaxation." *Archives of Internal Medicine,* 144, 1954-1958.

DeBakey, M. E., Gatto, A. M., & Foreyt, J. P. (1984). *The Living Heart Diet.* St. Louis: Fireside Books.

Fehr, L. A. (1983). *Introduction to Personality.* New York: Macmillan.

Fehr, L.A. (1992) "Theories of stress." In *Magill's Survey of Social Science: Psychology.* Salem Press Inc.

Fehr, L.A. (1988) "Effects of caffeine withdrawal on motor performance and heart rate changes." *International Journal of Psychophysiology,* 6, 9-14.

Friedman, M., & Rosenman, R. H. (1974). *Type-A Behavior And Your Heart.* New York: Knopf.

Friedman, M., & Ulmer, D. (1984). *Treating Type A Behavior And Your Heart.* New York: Knopf.

Gatchel, R. J., Baum, A., and Krantz, D. S. (1989). *An Introduction to Health Psychology (second edition).* New York: Random House.

Gill, J. L. (1983). "Personalized stress management." San Jose: *Counseling and Consulting Services Publications.*

Goleman, T., & Goleman, T. (1986). *The Relaxed Body Book.* New York: Doubleday & Co.

Glueck, C. J., Gordon, D. J., Nelson, J. J., Davis, J., &Tyroler, H. A. (1986). "Dietary and other correlates of changes in total and low density lipoprotein cholesterol in hypocholesterolemic men: The lipid research clinics coronary primary prevention trial." *American Journal of Clinical Nutrition,* 44, 489-500.

Gordon, T., Castelli, W. P., Hjortland, M. P., Kannel, W., & Dawber, T. R. (1977). "The Framingham study: High density lipoprotein as a protective factor against coronary heart disease." *American Journal of Medicine, 62,* 707-714.

Gottlieb, W., Lowe, C., Bricklin, M., and Zarrow, S. (1984). *The Complete Book of Vitamins.* Emmaus, PA: Rodale Press.

Greenberg, J. S. (1983). *Comprehensive Stress Management.* Dubuque, Iowa: W. C. Brown Publishers.

Hausman, P. (1984). *At a Glance Nutrition Counter.* New York: Ballantine Books.

Hegsted, D. M. (1986). "Serum-cholesterol response to dietary cholesterol: a re-evaluation." *American Journal of Clinical Nutrition,* 44, 299-305.

Hoffman, F. L. (1918). "The mortality from cancer in different occupations." Ztschr. d. osterr. Sanitatswesen, supplement to 1-26, pp. 33-42. *The Journal of Cancer Research, VI,* 4, 370-371.

Hoffman, S. A., Paschkis, K. E., DeBias, D. A., Cantarow, A., and Williams, T. L. (1961). "The influence

Vibrant Health

of exercise on the growth of transplanted rat tumors." *Cancer Research*, 22, 597-599.

Holmes, T. H., and Rahe, R. H. (1967). "The social readjustment rating scale." *Journal of Psychosomatic Research*, 11, 213-218.

Houston, M. C. (1986). "Review: Sodium and hypertension." *Archives of Internal Medicine*, 146, 179-185.

James, P. (1985). "Obesity: the interaction of environment and a genetic predisposition." In H. Trowell, D. Burkett, & K. Heaton (Eds.), *Dietary Fibre, Fibre-Depleted Foods and Disease*. New York: Academic Press, 249-261.

Jemmott, J. B., & Locke, S. E. (1984). "Psychosocial factors, immunologic meditation, and human susceptibility to infectious diseases: How much do we know?" *Psychological Bulletin*, 95, 52-77.

Keys, A. (1986). "Serum cholesterol response to dietary cholesterol." *American Journal of Clinical Nutrition*, 44, 309-311.

Kobasa, S. C. (1979) "Stressful life events, personality and health: An inquiry into hardiness." *Journal of Personality and Social Psychology* 39, 1-11.

Kowalski, R. E. (1988). *The 8-week Cholesterol Cure*. New York: Harper & Row.

Kritchevsky, D. (1985). "Lipid metabolism and coronary heart disease." In H. Trowell, D. Burkett, & K. Heaton (Eds.), *Dietary Fibre, Fibre-Depleted Foods and Disease*. New York: Academic Press, 305-315.

Krantz, D. S., Grunberg, N. E., & Baum, A. (1985). "Health Psychology." *Annual Review of Psychology*, 36, 349-383.

Lapidus, L., Andersson, H., Bengsston, C., & Bosaeus, I. (1986). "Dietary habits in relation to incidence of cardiovascular disease and death in women: a 12-year follow-up of participants in the population study of women in Gothenburg, Sweden." *American Journal of Clinical Nutrition, 44,* 444-448.

Larson, E. B., & Bruce, R. A. (1986). "Exercise and aging." Annals *of Internal Medicine,* 105, 5, 783-785.

Lazarus, R. S., & Folkman, S. (1984). *Stress, Appraisal and Coping.* New York: Springer.

LeShan, L. (1974). *How to Meditate.* New York: Bantam Books.

Lueg, M. C., & Anging, R. H. (1986). "Brief review: Hypercholesterolemia: new values, new strategies." *Hospital Practice,* Jan. 30, 112-121.

Mahoney, M. J., Moura, N. G. M., and Wade, T. C. "The relative efficacy of self-reward, self-punishment, and self-monitoring techniques for weight loss." *Journal of Consulting and Clinical Psychology,* 40, 404-407.

Matarazzo, J. D., Weiss, S. M., Herd, J. A., Miller, N. E., & Weiss, S. M. (Eds.). (1984). *Behavioral Health.* New York: Wiley.

Matthews, K. A. (1984). "Assessment of Type A, anger, and hostility in epidemiological studies of cardiovascular disease." In A. Ostfield & E. Eaker (Eds.), *Measuring Psychosocial Variables in Epidemiological Studies of Cardiovascular Disease.* Bethesda: National Institute of Health.

Michaud, El, Feinstein, A., Keough, C., and Feltman, J. (1989). *Fighting Disease: The Complete Guide to Natural Immune Power.* Emmaus, PA: Rodale Press.

Morehouse, L. E., & Miller, A. T. (1959). *Physiology of Exercise.* St. Louis: Mosby.

245

Nestel, P. J. (1986). "Fish oil attenuates the cholesterol induced rise in lipoprotein cholesterol." *American Journal of Clinical Nutrition*, 43, 752-757.

Oh, S. Y., & Miller, L. T. (1985). "Effect of dietary egg on variability of plasma cholesterol levels and lipoprotein cholesterol, 1-3." *American Journal of Clinical Nutrition*, 42, 421-431.

Oh, S. Y., & Monaco, P. A. (1985). "Effect of dietary cholesterol and degree of fat unsaturation on plasma lipid levels, lipoprotein composition and fecal steroid excretion in normal young adult men, 1-3." *American Journal of Clinical Nutrition*, 42, 399-413.

Ornish, D. (1983). *Stress, Diet and Your Heart.* New York: Holt, Rinehart & Winston.

Paffenbarger, R., Hyde, R., Wiag, L., & Steinmetz, C. (1984). "A natural history of athleticism and cardiovascular health." *Journal of the American Medical Association*, 252, 491-495.

Pauling, L. (1986). *How To Live Longer and Feel Better.* New York: Avon Books.

Polivy, J., & Herman, C. P. (1983). *Breaking the Diet Habit: The Natural Weight Alternative.* New York: Basic Books.

Powell, Drs. Tag & Judith (1991). *Silva Mind Mastery For The '90s.* Florida: Top Of The Mountain Publishing.

Roberts, H.J., M.D. (1992). *Sweet'ner Dearest: Bittersweet Vignettes About Aspartame (Nutrasweet®).* Florida: Sunshine Sentinel Press.

Rotter, J. B. (1966). "Generalized expectancies for internal versus external control of reinforcement." *Psychological Monographs*, 80.

Rubin, T. (1969). *The Angry Book*. New York: Macmillan.

Sady, S. P., Thompson, P. D., Cullinane, E. M., Kantor, M. A., Domagala, E., & Herbert, P. N. (1986). "Prolonged exercise augments plasma triglyceride clearance." *Journal of the American Medical Association*, 256, 18, 2552-2555.

Schachter, S. (1971). "Some extraordinary facts about obese humans and rats." *American Psychologist*, 26, 129-144.

Selye, H. (1956) *The Stress of Life*. New York: McGraw-Hill.

Selye, H. (1974). *Stress Without Distress*. Pennsylvania: Lippincott.

Sivertsen, I., and Dahlstrom, A.W. (1922). "The relation of muscular activity to carcinoma." *The Journal of Cancer Research*. VI, 4, 365-378.

Simko, V. (1978). "Physical exercise and the prevention of atherosclerosis and cholesterol gallstone." *Postgraduate Medical Journal*, 54, 828, 270-277.

Stamler, J., Wentworth, D., & Neaton, J. D. (1986). "Is the relationship between serum cholesterol and risk of premature death from coronary heart disease continuous and graded?" *Journal of the American Medical Association*, 256, 20, 2823-2827.

Stewart, C.T. (1990) "Anxiety: Theory, Assessment, and Management." Social *Science Perspectives Journal*, 4, 189-206.

Stewart, C.T. (1988). *Cancer: Prevention, Detection, Causes, Treatment*. Pennsylvania: Hampton Court Press.

Stewart, C.T. (1990) "Understanding and Managing Stress." *Proceedings of the Seventh Annual Conference of Academic Chairpersons*, 34, 334-344.

Zak, V., Carlin, C., & Vash, P. (1987). *The Fat-to-Muscle Diet*. New York: G. P. Putnam's Sons.

Zauner, C. W. (1985). "Physical fitness in aging men." *Maturitas*, 7, 267-271.

Index

Vibrant Health

Omega-3   43, 196
osteoporosis   81

P

Pauling, Linus   45
personality   105
  type A   110
    changing the   111
    characteristics of   109
    heart disease   110
    hostility   110
phobias. *See* fears
plan
  hard-easy principle   84
prayer   163
protein   34
  sources of   36

R

relaxation. *See also* stress
  reduction techniques

S

selenium   208
self-reward   129
soreness   99
sports   81
stress   136, 153
  aggression   141
  blood pressure   143
  death   145
  "fight or flight"   136
  illness   145
stress reduction techniques
  meditation
    mantra   164

modeling   171
stress reduction techniques
  attitude   161
  autogenic training   176
  being truthful   162
  biofeedback   173
    Menninger Foundation   174
    Raynaud's disease   174
  breathing   156
  drugs   154
  laughing   155
  meditation   163
  prayer   163
  progressive muscle relax-
    ation   165
  saying no   159
  soaking   158
  systematic desensitiza-
    tion   168
  walking   158
sugar
  substitutes
    Equal (aspartame)   32
    NutraSweet   32
    saccharine   32
    Sweet-n-Low   32
systematic desensitization
  modeling   171

T

thyroid   122

V

visualization   117
vitamins   43
  Vitamin A   44

Write, Call Or FAX For FREE Catalog

TOP OF THE MOUNTAIN PUBLISHING

11701 S. Belcher Road, Suite 123

Largo, Florida 34643-5117 U.S.A.

24-Hour FAX (813) 536-3681

Call (813) 530-0110